NEUROLOGY
FOR MRCP

The Essential Guide to Neurology for
MRCP Part 1, Part 2 and PACES

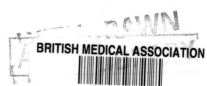

NEUROLOGY
FOR MRCP

The Essential Guide to Neurology for MRCP
Part 1, Part 2 and PACES

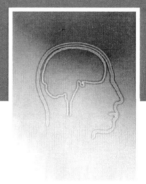

Jonathan D Rohrer
Jonathan Kennedy

UCL Institute of Neurology, Queen Square, UK

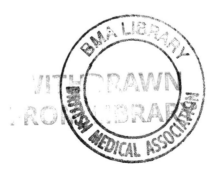

ICP

Imperial College Press

Published by

Imperial College Press
57 Shelton Street
Covent Garden
London WC2H 9HE

Distributed by

World Scientific Publishing Co. Pte. Ltd.
5 Toh Tuck Link, Singapore 596224
USA office: 27 Warren Street, Suite 401-402, Hackensack, NJ 07601
UK office: 57 Shelton Street, Covent Garden, London WC2H 9HE

British Library Cataloguing-in-Publication Data
A catalogue record for this book is available from the British Library.

Cover image: © Dr. Michael Miller & MTP Inc. Tokyo

NEUROLOGY FOR MRCP
The Essential Guide to Neurology for MRCP Part 1, Part 2 and PACES

Copyright © 2011 by Imperial College Press

ISBN-13 978-1-84816-462-8 (pbk)
ISBN-10 1-84816-462-9 (pbk)

Typeset by Stallion Press
Email: enquiries@stallionpress.com

Printed in Singapore.

Contents

List of Figures

Acknowledgements

We would like to thank Rebecca Miller and Fiona Kennedy for their support during the writing of the book.

We would also like to thank Dr Michael Miller for providing the cover design and Dr Edward Wild for kind permission to use the dermatomal map.

Lastly, we would also like to thank Dr Camilla Clark, Dr Lucy Reynolds and in particular Dr Phillip Kennedy for reviewing the manuscript.

Introduction

Neurology is commonly portrayed as a difficult topic in the MRCP examinations. This book has been written to try and help you through both the written and clinical sections of the exam and hopefully prove that Neurology is not as difficult as it may at first seem. The book is not designed, however, to be a definitive Neurology textbook but rather a revision guide for the MRCP exams.

The first section of the book describes the neurological disorders you need to know about for the MRCP and will be useful throughout the different parts of the exam. The second section of the book concentrates on the PACES section of the exam. The third section provides questions to test your knowledge before the Part 1 and Part 2 exams. Each section is set out in roughly anatomical fashion, starting with disorders of the cortex and moving down through the nervous system to finish at the muscle. This systematic way of thinking is useful for both the written and clinical exam and will be used as the basis for the book.

It is important to recognise that in practice, different neurologists may all perform the neurological examination slightly differently and in their own idiosyncratic way. For PACES it is advisable to perform a standard 'textbook' neurological examination as set out in Section 2 of this book.

Dr Jonathan Rohrer
MRCP (UK)

Dr Jonathan Kennedy
MRCP (UK)

Part 1
Neurological Disorders

Chapter 1

Basic Anatomy

The Cortex

The cerebral hemispheres have an outer layer, the cortex, which consists of grey matter and surrounds the inner white matter. The cortex is intricately folded with the convolutions or ridges called gyri and the fissures in between called sulci. The important sulci to remember are:

- The longitudinal fissure which separates the two hemispheres.
- The lateral (or Sylvian) fissure which separates the frontal and parietal lobes superiorly from the temporal lobe inferiorly.
- The central sulcus which separates the frontal lobe from the parietal lobe.

In the vast majority of people (virtually all right-handers and around 70% of left-handers) the left hemisphere is 'dominant' for language.

Each of the frontal, temporal, parietal and occipital lobes has specific functions:

Frontal lobe

- Executive function, e.g. planning or decision making
- Behaviour
- Speech production (Broca's area) — dominant hemisphere
- Motor cortex

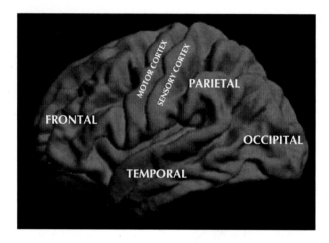

Fig. 1. Cerebral hemisphere showing the frontal, temporal, parietal and occipital lobes.

Temporal lobe

- Episodic memory (medial temporal lobe)
- Semantic memory
- Speech comprehension (Wernicke's area) — dominant hemisphere
- Auditory cortex

Parietal lobe

- Dominant hemisphere: calculation, reading, writing, limb praxis
- Non-dominant hemisphere: visuospatial/visuoperceptual skills
- Sensory cortex

Occipital lobe

- Visual cortex

Basal Ganglia

The basal ganglia are a group of deep grey matter nuclei: caudate, putamen, globus pallidus, substantia nigra and subthalamic nucleus.

They have a number of roles but the key group of neurological disorders associated with the basal ganglia are the movement disorders.

Cerebellum

The cerebellum consists of two hemispheres joined in the middle by the vermis.

It is involved in motor control and damage leads to problems with coordination ipsilateral to the side of the lesion.

Cranial Nerves

There are 12 cranial nerves. The olfactory (1st) and optic (2nd) nerves pass straight into the brain but the nuclei for cranial nerves 3 to 12 are situated in the brainstem and can be roughly split into:

- Midbrain: oculomotor (3rd), trochlear (4th)
- Pons: trigeminal (5th), abducens (6th), facial (7th) and vestibulo-cochlear (8th)
- Medulla: glossopharyngeal (9th), vagus (10th), accessory (11th) and hypoglosssal (12th).

This is a rough division as the sensory nuclei for the 5th nerve extend throughout the brainstem. The nuclei are either medial or lateral in the brainstem:

Medial: 3rd, 4th, 6th and 12th (i.e. those that are factors of 12)
Lateral: 5th, 7th, 8th, 9th, 10th, 11th

This basic cranial nerve anatomy is useful when identifying the cranial nerves that will be affected by lesions occurring at various points in the brainstem (e.g. the lateral medulla).

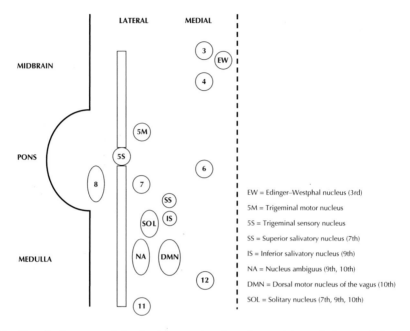

Fig. 2. A diagram of the brainstem showing the position of the cranial nerve nuclei.

Motor Pathway

The motor pathway starts in the motor cortex with the upper motor neurone travelling down the corticospinal tract laterally in the brainstem, crossing to the opposite side in the medulla and down the spinal cord where it synapses with the lower motor neurone in the anterior horn. The lower motor neurone travels through the spinal roots, plexus then nerve to synapse with the muscle at the neuro-muscular junction.

Sensory Pathway

Sensation is carried from receptors via sensory nerves, the plexus and roots to the spinal cord where it ascends in two main tracts: the spinothalamic tract which is anterior in the cord and carries pain and temperature sense, and the dorsal columns which is posterior in the

Upper Limb Movement	Roots	Nerves	Muscles
Shoulder abduction	C5	Axillary	Deltoid
Shoulder adduction	C6/C7	Lateral/medial pectoral	Pectoralis major
		Thoracodorsal	Latissimus dorsi
		Lower subscapular	Teres major
Elbow extension	C7/C8	Radial	Triceps
Elbow flexion (supinated)	C5/C6	Musculocutaneous	Biceps
Elbow flexion (mid-prone)	C5/C6	Radial	Brachioradialis
Wrist extension	C6	Radial	Extensor carpi radialis
	C7	Posterior interosseous	Extensor carpi ulnaris
Wrist flexion	C6/C7	Median	Flexor carpi radialis
	C8	Ulnar	Flexor carpi ulnaris
Finger extension	C7	Posterior interosseous	Extensor digitorum, indicis and digiti minimi
Finger flexion (MCP joints)	C8/T1	Median/ulnar	Lumbricals
	C8/T1	Ulnar	Flexor digiti minimi
Finger flexion (PIP joints)	C8	Median	Flexor digitorum superficialis
Finger flexion (DIP joints)	C8	Anterior interosseous/ulnar	Flexor digitorum profundus
Finger abduction	T1	Ulnar	Dorsal interossei
	C8/T1	Ulnar	Abductor digiti minimi
Finger adduction	T1	Ulnar	Palmar interossei
Thumb abduction	T1	Median	Abductor pollicis brevis

Lower Limb Movement	Roots	Nerves	Muscles
Hip flexion	L1/L2/L3	Femoral, Branches from L1-3	Iliopsoas
Hip extension	L5/S1	Inferior gluteal	Gluteus maximus
Hip abduction	L4/L5/S1	Superior gluteal	Gluteus medius/minimus
Hip adduction	L2/L3/L4	Obturator	Adductors
Knee flexion	L5/S1	Sciatic	Hamstrings
Knee extension	L3/L4	Femoral	Quadriceps
Ankle dorsiflexion	L4/L5	Deep peroneal	Tibialis anterior
Ankle plantarflexion	S1/S2	Tibial	Gastrocnemius, soleus
Foot inversion	L4/L5	Tibial	Tibialis posterior
Foot eversion	L5/S1	Superficial peroneal	Peroneus longus/brevis
Big toe extension	L5	Deep peroneal	Extensor hallucis longus

cord and carries vibration sense and proprioception (joint position sense). Light touch is carried by both tracts. The spinothalamic tract crosses to the other side (decussates) almost as soon as it enters the spinal cord whilst the dorsal columns do not cross until the medulla. Neurones in both tracts synapse in the thalamus with the final neurone passing from there through the internal capsule to the sensory cortex.

It is important to remember the dermatomal sensory representation:

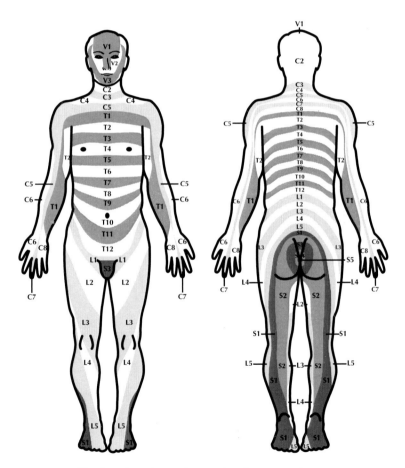

Fig. 3. Anterior and posterior dermatomal map.

Chapter 2

Dementia and Delirium

Dementia

This is defined as an acquired, progressive impairment of cognition that interferes with social functioning.

It usually occurs in the older age group. The majority of patients have either a neurodegenerative disease or cerebrovascular disease but it is important to rule out rare 'reversible' causes. Four diseases account for around 95% of patients with dementia:

- Alzheimer's disease (~60%)
- Vascular dementia (~20%)
- Dementia with Lewy bodies (~10%)
- Frontotemporal dementia (~5%)

Alzheimer's Disease (AD)

- It usually presents with amnestic symptoms — loss of episodic and topographical memory. The disease progresses to global cognitive impairment.
- Genetically, ApoE4 is a risk factor but autosomal dominant AD is rare and is due to mutations in APP, presenilin 1 or presenilin 2.
- Abnormal proteins found pathologically are amyloid (plaques) and tau (neurofibrillary tangles). Acetylcholine is deficient.
- Rarely, pathological AD can present with non-amnestic symptoms, e.g. with biparietal features (posterior cortical atrophy) or with language impairment (logopenic aphasia).

Vascular Dementia (VaD)

- VaD has similar risk factors to other cerebrovascular disease.
- Slowing of thinking (bradyphrenia) may be the dominant feature.
- Most patients will have a progressive history rather than the classical stepwise progression of 'multi-infarct' dementia.
- As age is a risk factor for both AD and VaD, many patients will have a mixed dementia with features of both.

Dementia with Lewy Bodies (DLB)

- DLB presents with parkinsonism, cognitive impairment (which may fluctuate), visual hallucinations, REM sleep disorder and neuroleptic sensitivity.
- The abnormal protein found pathologically (in Lewy bodies) is alpha-synuclein. Dopamine and acetylcholine are deficient.
- Patients with Parkinson's disease can develop a similar dementia many years into the illness: Parkinson's disease dementia (PDD).

Frontotemporal Dementia (FTD)

- This is a heterogeneous group of disorders including behavioural variant FTD (formerly Pick's disease), semantic dementia and progressive non-fluent aphasia.
- It overlaps with progressive supranuclear palsy and corticobasal degeneration, as well as motor neurone disease.
- Behavioural variant FTD presents with a change in personality, e.g. disinhibition, loss of empathy and/or apathy. Apart from executive dysfunction, other cognitive domains are usually intact early on.
- Abnormal proteins found pathologically are tau, TDP-43 or FUS.

- Genetically, up to 50% of cases are familial with the most common mutations in the tau and progranulin genes (which are autosomal dominant).

The other 5% of cases of dementia are accounted for by many different diseases:

- Neurodegenerative: Huntington's disease, prion disease
- Inflammation/infection: cerebral vasculitis, MS, HIV, SLE, neurosyphilis
- Metabolic/toxic: vitamin B12 deficiency, chronic alcohol use, Wilson's disease, hypothyroidism
- Other: normal pressure hydrocephalus (a triad of dementia, impaired gait and urinary incontinence)

Prion Disease

- Sporadic Creutzfeldt–Jakob disease (CJD): rapidly progressive dementia with myoclonus and cerebellar syndrome. EEG shows periodic sharp wave complexes, CSF is positive for 14-3-3 protein, MRI shows signal change in the basal ganglia.
- Variant CJD: only around 200 definite cases have ever been described worldwide at present and all with the same prion protein gene MM genotype at codon 129. It usually presents in a younger age group (average age at onset of late 20s) with early psychiatric and sensory symptoms followed by dementia, myoclonus and a cerebellar syndrome. MRI shows signal change in the thalamus ('pulvinar sign').
- Prion disease can also be familial due to a mutation in the prion protein gene.

Investigations

- Blood tests: TFTs, vitamin B12, ANA, ENA, syphilis serology; rarely, genetic testing is performed.
- Brain scan (CT or MRI): exclude structural lesions mimicking dementia, e.g. tumours or chronic subdural haematoma, and help to make a diagnosis, e.g. MRI to look for hippocampal atrophy in AD.
- Other investigations in specific circumstances include lumbar puncture, EEG and neuropsychology testing.

Management

- There is no curative treatment for the neurodegenerative dementias.
- Symptomatic treatment with the cholinesterase inhibitors (donepezil, rivastigmine and galantamine) has some benefit in both AD and DLB. In the UK, their use is currently limited by NICE guidelines (AD patients must score 10–20 on the MMSE).
- Side effects of the cholinesterase inhibitors include gastrointestinal symptoms and urinary frequency. They can cause cardiac conduction abnormalities and should not be used in patients with 2nd or 3rd degree heart block.

Delirium (Acute Confusional State)

This is defined as disturbance of attention, concentration and orientation with onset over hours to days and fluctuations over the day. Causes include:

- Metabolic/electrolyte abnormalities, e.g. hypoglycaemia, hypercalcaemia, liver disease (hepatic encephalopathy), uraemia, hyponatraemia, hypothyroidism
- Infections, e.g. urinary tract, chest
- Neurological disorders, e.g. stroke, meningitis/encephalitis, post-seizure
- Drugs/toxins, e.g. alcohol
- Hypoxia

Patients with dementia are more prone to become acutely confused.

Wernicke's Encephalopathy

- This is due to thiamine (vitamin B1) deficiency often in association with chronic alcohol use or repeated vomiting.
- There is a triad of features of acute confusion, a cerebellar syndrome (ataxia) and an eye movement disorder (most commonly nystagmus but a 6th nerve palsy or internuclear ophthalmoplegia can occur).
- Anatomically, the mamillary bodies, thalamus, midbrain and cerebellum are affected.
- Red cell transketolase level is reduced.
- Intravenous thiamine should be given. Patients should not be given a glucose load before treatment as this may worsen the symptoms.
- Irreversible damage may occur leading to a permanent amnesic syndrome (Korsakoff syndrome).

Chapter 3

Epilepsy

This is a disorder characterized by a tendency to have recurrent seizures, i.e. abnormal cerebral electrical activity.

Classification of Seizures

A. *Partial — onset localised to a focal area of the brain*

1. Simple (consciousness unimpaired)
2. Complex (consciousness impaired)
3. Secondarily generalised

B. *Generalised*

1. Absence ('petit mal')
   They occur mostly in childhood, consisting of short-lived episodes of unawareness (usually less than 30 seconds) where the patient may look blank and stare, with return to normal straight after the episode.
2. Tonic-clonic ('grand mal')
   These occur without warning. There is loss of consciousness and the limbs become stiff (tonic phase) followed by convulsive movements of the limbs (clonic phase). There may be tongue biting and/or urinary incontinence. Apnoea also occurs and the patient may become cyanosed. A post-ictal period follows, often lasting hours, where the patient feels fatigued, confused and may have a headache.

3. Myoclonic
4. Tonic
5. Clonic
6. Atonic

Investigations

The diagnosis of a seizure is based largely on an informant history and may be supported by investigations:

- ECG should be performed. A 24-hour tape may be necessary if it is unclear whether the event is a seizure or is related to an arrhythmia, i.e. cardiac syncope.
- With a suspected seizure, blood tests should be performed, including the measurement of electrolytes, calcium and magnesium.
- Interictal routine EEG will be normal in around half of patients with epilepsy. Sensitivity improves with longer recordings, hyperventilation and with sleep-deprived EEG.
- Brain scan (CT or preferably MRI) should be performed.

Management

Treatment with an anti-epileptic drug (AED) usually occurs following two or more seizures. The most commonly used first-line AEDs are carbamazepine (first line for partial seizures), sodium valproate and lamotrigine. Other drugs used include levetiracetam and topiramate. Phenytoin is now used mainly in status epilepticus. Many patients will only require monotherapy but some will require multiple AEDs. Side effects of the main drugs include:

- Sodium valproate: nausea/vomiting, tremor, weight gain, alopecia, polycystic ovaries, hyperammonaemia, teratogenicity, parkinsonism

- Carbamazepine: dizziness, rash, neutropaenia, SIADH
- Lamotrigine: rash, Stevens–Johnson syndrome
- Phenytoin: cerebellar syndrome (in toxicity), acne, hirsutism, gum hypertrophy, facial coarsening, peripheral neuropathy, osteomalacia

Carbamazepine and phenytoin are enzyme inducers whilst sodium valproate is an enzyme inhibitor.

Advice to patients with epilepsy:

- *Driving* — patients must contact the DVLA. Patients with a diagnosis of epilepsy can drive again after one year of being seizure-free or after three years if their seizures occur only during sleep. If a patient has only had a single seizure however, they can drive again after six months if investigations (EEG/brain scan) are normal. HGV and passenger-carrying vehicle drivers must be seizure-free for ten years.
- *Contraception* — women taking an enzyme-inducing AED will need to take a higher dose of the oral contraceptive pill.
- *Pregnancy* — many of the drugs have a risk of teratogenicity and this is higher in valproate (which can cause neural tube defects) than in lamotrigine or carbamazepine. Women considering conceiving should take regular folate (5 mg per day).
- *Safety measures* — patients should not bathe or swim alone and should not take part in any sports considered dangerous.

Status Epilepticus

This occurs when a patient has a seizure or series of seizures lasting longer than 30 minutes without regaining consciousness. A treatment pathway for status epilepticus is as follows:

- Basic life support
- Early status: IV lorazepam (if no IV access, diazepam can be given rectally)

- Established status: IV phenytoin or fosphenytoin +/– IV phenobarbitone
- Refractory status: involve the ICU team — intubate and use propofol, thiopentone or midazolam

Juvenile Myoclonic Epilepsy

- This is an epileptic disorder that starts in childhood, often with a family history.
- Upper limb myoclonic jerks occur as well as tonic-clonic seizures (often arising from sleep) and in some patients there may be absence seizures.
- Carbamazepine should be avoided as this worsens the myoclonus.

Temporal Lobe Epilepsy (TLE)

- This is the most common cause of partial seizures, usually causing complex partial seizures, i.e. with impaired consciousness.
- The origin is usually hippocampal with hippocampal sclerosis being the underlying cause.
- Prior to the seizure there may be an aura. Symptoms include a rising feeling in the stomach, olfactory or gustatory hallucinations, déjà vu, a sense of fear and a feeling of depersonalisation.
- Impaired consciousness then occurs often with automatisms such as lip smacking, chewing or fidgeting.
- Patients are then confused post-ictally.
- TLE can cause the syndrome of transient epileptic amnesia (TEA) where patients have recurrent episodes of memory impairment.

Non-Epileptic Attack Disorder

- Dissociative or psychogenic seizures can occur. They can be difficult to distinguish from true seizures but pointers to a dissociative seizure include closed eyelids with resistance to eye opening, biting the tip (rather than the side) of the tongue, undulating motor activity, asynchronous limb movements, side-to-side head shaking, lack of cyanosis, rapid post-ictal orientation and regular lengthy seizures.
- Dissociative seizures may occur at times in people who also have epilepsy, i.e. true seizures.
- Video telemetry (continuous EEG monitoring whilst being videoed) can be useful in diagnosing dissociative seizures.

Chapter 4

Raised Intracranial Pressure

This usually presents with a headache which is postural, i.e. worse first thing in the morning, after lying flat or bending forwards and worse on straining or coughing (which increase pressure further). Other symptoms may be nausea/vomiting and visual symptoms (obscurations, diplopia) or, if severe, a drop in consciousness level. Papilloedema (which may lead to an enlarged blind spot) is seen on fundoscopic examination.

Causes include:

- Space-occupying lesions (e.g. tumours, abscesses)
- Idiopathic intracranial hypertension
- Cerebral venous sinus thrombosis
- Head injury
- Hydrocephalus (increased amount of CSF in the brain)

Brain Tumors

- Symptoms include seizures, features of raised intracranial pressure and focal neurological deficits.
- The most common brain tumours are metastases from a carcinoma elsewhere in the body. These may present before there are symptoms from the primary.
- Primary brain tumours include gliomas, i.e. astrocytomas, oligodendrogliomas and ependymomas: grades 1 and 2 are

said to be 'benign' whilst grades 3 and 4 are 'malignant', including glioblastoma multiforme (a grade 4 tumour).

- Other benign tumours include meningiomas, pituitary tumours and acoustic neuromas (vestibular schwannomas).
- Cerebral lymphoma can occur, with an increased incidence in the immunocompromised.

Idiopathic ('Benign') Intracranial Hypertension

- This occurs more commonly in young overweight people, with a greater incidence in females. It is associated with oral contraceptive use as well as other drug use: tetracyclines, vitamin A, retinoids, nitrofurantoin, lithium.
- Clinical features are those of raised intracranial pressure.
- An MRI brain scan is performed to exclude another cause of raised intracranial pressure (e.g. space-occupying lesion or venous sinus thrombosis). Lumbar puncture should then be performed to measure the opening pressure (>25 cm H_2O).
- Any causative drug should be stopped and patients advised to lose weight. Acetazolamide is used as a first-line diuretic, although some patients may need repeated lumbar punctures. In severe cases (e.g. when vision becomes impaired) a shunt (ventriculo-peritoneal or lumbo-peritoneal) may be necessary.

Chapter 5

Cerebrovascular Disease

A stroke is a sudden onset focal neurological deficit, secondary to cerebrovascular disease, lasting more than 24 hours. Traditionally, a transient ischaemic attack (TIA) is defined as an episode lasting less than 24 hours. Strokes occur due to either ischaemia (about 85%) or haemorrhage.

Ischaemia

Most ischaemic strokes are due to thrombosis or embolism. The commonest cause is atherosclerosis (large vessel more frequently than small vessel disease) with the main risk factors being hypertension, hypercholesterolaemia, smoking and diabetes mellitus. Embolism from the heart is also a common cause, with the major risk factor being atrial fibrillation but other risk factors include valvular disease, artificial heart valves, recent myocardial infarction, endocarditis and cardiac tumours. Other causes of ischaemic strokes include:

- Arterial (e.g. carotid or vertebral) dissection
- Vasculitis
- Haematological disorders: polycythaemia, thrombocythaemia, sickle cell disease, antiphospholipid syndrome, leukaemia
- Genetic disorders: CADASIL, MELAS
- Recreational drug use: cocaine, amphetamine

Ischaemia can also be caused by hypoperfusion of the brain leading to so-called 'watershed' or border zone infarcts.

Occasionally, strokes are caused by venous disease, either due to cerebral venous sinus thrombosis or by paradoxical embolism in a patient with an atrial septal defect or patent foramen ovale.

Haemorrhage

Intracerebral haemorrhage is usually associated with chronic hypertension in patients with small vessel disease but less commonly may be caused by other conditions including anticoagulant use, amyloid angiopathy, cavernomas, arteriovenous malformations and aneurysms.

Treatment

All patients should be scanned within the first 24 hours (and preferably as soon as possible) with either a CT or MRI brain scan. MRI scanning with diffusion weighted imaging can identify whether a stroke is acute.

For ischaemic strokes:

- Intravenous thrombolysis with tissue plasminogen activator (tPA) can be given if patients fit local criteria and present within 4.5 hours.
- Following thrombolysis or first-line treatment if not thrombolysed, most patients will receive antiplatelet therapy with

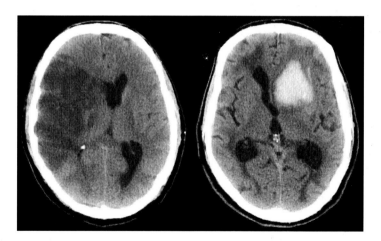

Fig. 4. CT scans showing a left middle cerebral artery infarction (on the left) and right hemisphere intracerebral haemorrhage (on the right).

aspirin +/– dipyridamole. Patients who cannot take aspirin can use clopidogrel.
- In specific cases (particularly cardioembolic stroke), anticoagulation is used. In patients with atrial fibrillation, warfarin is started 10–14 days after the stroke.

For all patients:
- Treatment within a dedicated stroke unit improves outcome.
- Rehabilitation with physiotherapy, occupational therapy and speech therapy.
- Nutrition is important and nasogastric tube placement is necessary if a patient's swallow is affected. PEG may be required in the long-term.
- Vascular risk factor management — smoking cessation, statins for hypercholesterolaemia, blood pressure management, diabetic control.
- Carotid Doppler studies — if patients have greater than 70% (and less than 100%) stenosis of the carotid artery on the symptomatic side then they are candidates for carotid endarterectomy.
- Echocardiogram can be useful to identify cardiac thrombus.
- 24-hour tape can identify paroxysmal atrial fibrillation.

Stroke can be classified in different ways. One common method is the Oxfordshire Community Stroke Project classification which defines four groups: TACI (total anterior circulation infarct), PACI (partial anterior circulation infarct), POCI (posterior circulation infarct) and LACI (lacunar infarct). Symptoms and signs of strokes depend on the territory of the brain affected.

Anterior circulation (carotid territory) infarct

Ophthalmic artery

- Monocular visual loss (in a TIA this is known as amaurosis fugax)

Middle cerebral artery

- Contralateral hemiparesis (face and arm > leg)

- Contralateral hemisensory loss
- Homonymous hemianopia
- Neglect
- Aphasia (dominant hemisphere): Broca's ('expressive'/nonfluent), Wernicke's ('receptive'/fluent) or global

Anterior cerebral artery

- Contralateral hemiparesis (leg > arm)

Posterior circulation (vertebrobasilar territory) infarct

Posterior cerebral artery

- Contralateral homonymous hemianopia (which may be macular-sparing, as this may be supplied by the middle cerebral artery)

Posterior inferior cerebellar artery (Lateral medullary syndrome)

- Contralateral impairment of pain/temperature sensation in the limb with ipsilateral impairment of pain/temperature in the face
- Ipsilateral Horner's syndrome
- Ipsilateral cerebellar signs, dysarthria, vertigo, vomiting, dysphagia

Other brainstem stroke syndromes

- Apart from the lateral medullary syndrome, other brainstem stroke syndromes are rare, e.g. the medial medullary syndrome which causes ipsilateral tongue weakness and contralateral hemiparesis in the arm and leg.

Lacunar Infarct

Small penetrating arteries to basal ganglia, thalamus, pons, internal capsule

- Most commonly a contralateral hemiparesis, contralateral hemisensory disturbance or both, without any cortical signs. Other syndromes seen include ataxic hemiparesis and dysarthria-clumsy hand.

Carotid Dissection

- This is a common cause of young-onset stroke and may occur spontaneously or following neck trauma.
- Clinical features are ipsilateral neck pain and/or headache (although these may be absent) followed by a focal neurological deficit. In many people an ipsilateral Horner's syndrome will be present.
- MRI scan with fat-suppressed T1-weighted images of the neck are used in the diagnosis. Patients should be anticoagulated.

CADASIL

- Cerebral autosomal dominant arteriopathy with subcortical infarcts and leucoencephalopathy (CADASIL) is a rare genetic disorder caused by mutations in the notch 3 gene. Patients may have associated migraine.

Watershed (Border Zone) Infarcts

- These are caused by hypoperfusion of the brain due to any cause, e.g. cardiac arrest or during cardiopulmonary bypass.
- The most susceptible areas are those at the border zone between different arterial territories, e.g. between anterior and middle cerebral arteries or between middle and posterior cerebral arteries.
- Bilateral watershed infarcts affecting the border zone between anterior and middle cerebral arteries cause bilateral proximal arm weakness (the 'man in the barrel').

Cerebral Venous Sinus Thrombosis

- Venous thrombosis initially leads to raised intracranial pressure and hence headache with papilloedema.

Subsequently infarction or haemorrhage may occur, leading to focal neurological signs. Seizures may also occur.

- Evidence of a venous thrombosis may be seen on CT, but MRI with MR venography is usually used in diagnosis. Patients should be anticoagulated.

Subarachnoid Haemorrhage (SAH)

- SAH is caused by the rupture of an intracranial 'berry' aneurysm in the majority of cases. Other causes include arteriovenous malformations.
- Clinical features are of a sudden onset severe 'thunderclap' headache with nausea and vomiting. Other features include meningism (stiff neck and photophobia, due to irritation of the meninges by blood), focal neurological signs and seizures.
- Complications include rebleeding, hydrocephalus, delayed ischaemia and hyponatraemia due to SIADH.
- SAH is usually seen on CT scan particularly if scanned early. However if SAH is still likely in the presence of a negative scan then a lumbar puncture to look for xanthochromia should be performed. This will be positive between about 12 hours and two weeks.
- Initial supportive measures are important. Nimodipine is given to prevent vasospasm and hence delayed ischaemia. Angiography is then necessary to identify the underlying abnormality. Coiling (endovascularly) or clipping (neurosurgically) can be used to treat aneurysms.

Chapter 6

Headache

Acute Headache

This is an important medical emergency and causes include:

- CNS infections: meningitis, encephalitis
- Vascular disease: subarachnoid haemorrhage, other intracranial haemorrhage, ischaemic stroke, arterial dissection, vasculitis, cerebral venous sinus thrombosis
- Other intracranial disease: raised intracranial pressure, low intracranial pressure (including post-lumbar puncture), pituitary apoplexy
- Primary headache syndromes: migraine, trigeminal autonomic cephalgias
- Non-neurological conditions: acute glaucoma, sinusitis, non-cranial infections, drugs

Patients need an urgent CT scan followed by lumbar puncture in most cases.

Primary Headache Syndromes

The most common types of headache are episodic:

- migraine
- trigeminal autonomic cephalgias, e.g. cluster headache, paroxysmal hemicrania
- tension headache (a featureless headache, i.e. no other symptoms)

They can become daily in occurrence (chronic daily headache) which may be associated with analgesia overuse.

Migraine

- This is a common episodic headache syndrome. Pain is throbbing, often unilateral and made worse by movement, light (photophobia) and sound (phonophobia). There may be associated nausea and vomiting. Episodes last four to 72 hours.
- Aura occur in around 20% of patients and consist of visual disturbances (e.g. flashes of lights or zigzag lines in front of the eyes), paraesthesia or other neurological symptoms.
- Treatment may be only of the acute episodes with simple analgesia (e.g. aspirin) or a triptan but if there are greater than three episodes a month then prophylaxis is used (e.g. propranolol, pizotifen, amitriptyline, sodium valproate, topiramate).

Cluster Headache

- Headaches are retro-orbital and unilateral, lasting for 15 minutes to three hours, occurring in clusters (e.g. for weeks at a time) with intervening pain-free periods. Patients are usually restless during an attack. Associated autonomic features are seen and include ipsilateral conjunctival injection, lacrimation, nasal congestion, rhinorrhoea and Horner's syndrome (ptosis and miosis).
- Simple analgesia may not be helpful acutely and triptans or 100% oxygen can be used. Prophylaxis, e.g. with verapamil, may be necessary.

Chapter 7

Neuroinfectious Disease

Acute Meningitis

This usually presents with an acute severe headache and fever with features of 'meningism', i.e. photophobia and neck stiffness. If it is severe, there may be confusion or decreased levels of consciousness. A non-blanching rash may be seen in patients with meningococcal meningitis.

- Bacterial: meningococcal (*Neisseria meningitidis*), pneumococcal (*Streptococcus pneumoniae*), *Haemophilus influenzae*, *Listeria monocytogenes*, *Staphylococcus aureus* and Gram-negative rods (e.g. *Escherichia coli*)
- Viral: enteroviruses, herpes viruses

Most patients will initially have a CT brain scan and this is then followed by a lumbar puncture. CSF should be sent to microbiology for an urgent cell count and Gram stain, and to biochemistry for protein and glucose measurement (with a matched serum glucose sample). CSF is usually also sent to virology, cytology and in certain circumstances for other specific tests (e.g. for TB and *Cryptococcus* when the history is more subacute).

It is important to give early antibiotic treatment (and not delay for the investigations), usually with a third-generation cephalosporin. If *Listeria* is suspected, then the patient should also receive ampicillin.

Subacute and Chronic Meningitis

This is unusual in an immunocompetent patient and more commonly occurs in the immunocompromised, e.g. patients with HIV infection. Headache and fever present subacutely and may be associated with a non-specific lethargy and malaise. Infective causes include TB, *Cryptococcus neoformans*, Lyme disease and syphilis. For TB, Ziehl–Neelsen staining and TB PCR of CSF are usually performed as well as a culture. For *Cryptococcus*, India ink stain can be positive, but serum and CSF cryptococcal antigen testing is more sensitive.

Non-infective causes of a chronic meningitis include sarcoidosis and neoplastic disease (e.g. lymphomatous or carcinomatous meningitis).

Encephalitis

Infective encephalitis presents with fever and confusion. Conscious level may be decreased and seizures can occur. It is usually viral in origin, and in the UK it will most commonly be caused by herpes simplex virus (HSV) and enteroviruses. Outside the UK, other causes include Japanese encephalitis virus and West Nile virus. Empirical treatment in the UK is with aciclovir for presumed HSV disease.

Lyme Disease

This is caused by *Borrelia* infection transmitted by tick bite. Neurological manifestations include cranial neuropathies, e.g. 7th nerve palsy, radiculopathy, neuropathy and chronic meningoencephalitis.

Protozoal Infections

- Toxoplasmosis (*Toxoplasma gondii*) causes ring-enhancing cerebral lesions and presents as headaches, seizures and focal neurological deficits.

- Cerebral malaria (*Plasmodium falciparum* spread by the Anopheles mosquito) can cause encephalopathy with decreased consciousness and seizures.
- African trypanosomiasis (*Trypanosoma brucei* spread by the tsetse fly) can cause a chronic meningoencephalitis leading to apathy and the tendency to fall asleep ('sleeping sickness').

Helminthic Infections

- Cysticercosis is caused by larvae of the *Taenia solium* tapeworm and leads to seizures with multiple lesions seen on MR imaging.

HIV

A variety of neurological disorders can occur in HIV-positive patients:

- HIV itself can cause encephalopathy/dementia, myelopathy and neuropathy.
- Opportunistic infections include toxoplasmosis, cryptococcal meningitis, CMV encephalitis and TB meningitis.
- Progressive multifocal leucoencephalopathy (PML) is due to infection by JC virus and causes headache, focal neurological deficits and seizures. MRI shows asymmetrical signal change in the white matter.
- Cerebral lymphoma usually presents with headache, focal neurological deficits and seizures as well as lethargy and confusion.

Chapter 8

Movement Disorders

Movement disorders are usually split into those resulting in too little movement, i.e. those with bradykinesia and rigidity (**akinetic-rigid syndromes**) and those causing too much movement (**hyperkinesias** or **dyskinesias**). Dyskinesias can either be:

a) jerky in nature, i.e. myoclonus, tics and chorea (including ballism) or
b) not jerky, i.e. tremor and dystonia (including athetosis).

Akinetic-Rigid Syndromes

Although the following disorders are classified under the akinetic-rigid (or extrapyramidal, or parkinsonian) syndromes, they usually have more than just bradykinesia and rigidity, e.g. in Parkinson's disease there is also tremor present.

Causes

- Parkinson's disease
- Drugs: neuroleptics, some antiemetics (e.g. metoclopramide), sodium valproate
- Other neurodegenerative diseases: progressive supranuclear palsy, corticobasal degeneration, multiple system atrophy, dementia with Lewy bodies
- Toxic: manganese, carbon monoxide
- Vascular disease
- Other: Wilson's disease, post-encephalitic

Parkinson's Disease (PD)

- The classic triad of clinical features are bradykinesia, rigidity and a rest tremor, which are initially asymmetrical. Postural instability is also seen.
- Non-motor features include sleep and neuropsychiatric disorders (e.g. depression and dementia) and autonomic dysfunction (e.g. GI or urinary problems).
- The diagnosis of PD is based on clinical features, but can be supported by abnormal dopamine transporter imaging (^{123}I-FP-CIT SPECT scan, also known as a DaTSCAN).
- The abnormal protein found pathologically is alpha-synuclein.
- Dopamine is deficient neurochemically.
- Initial treatment is with a dopamine agonist (ropinirole or pramipexole) or levodopa (with a DOPA-decarboxylase inhibitor). Agonists are usually the first treatment in younger patients. Side effects include nausea, hypotension, visual hallucinations and (particularly with dopamine agonists) impulse control disorders (repetitive obsessive behaviours) such as overusing medication, pathological gambling, hypersexuality and compulsive eating.
- Chronic use of levodopa is associated with dyskinesias, wearing-off effects towards the end of each dose and on-off fluctuations.
- Other drugs used are MAO inhibitors, e.g. selegiline or rasagiline, COMT inhibitors, e.g. entacapone, amantadine and apomorphine.
- Some severely affected patients benefit from deep brain stimulation.

Progressive Supranuclear Palsy (PSP)

- This usually presents with backward falls and there is a gaze palsy (initially vertical) and axial rigidity on examination.

- There is an overlap with frontotemporal dementia — patients may have behavioural symptoms and/or cognitive impairment.
- The abnormal protein found pathologically is tau.
- There is a poor response to levodopa.

Corticobasal Degeneration (CBD)

- This usually presents with an asymmetrical akinetic-rigid syndrome with dystonia, myoclonus and limb apraxia. An 'alien limb' phenomenon may be present.
- There is an overlap with frontotemporal dementia — patients may have behavioural symptoms, aphasia and/or cognitive impairment.
- The abnormal protein found pathologically is most commonly tau.
- There is a poor response to levodopa.

Multiple System Atrophy (MSA)

- This is a combination of an akinetic-rigid syndrome, cerebellar syndrome and autonomic dysfunction.
- If an akinetic-rigid syndrome predominates, it is known as MSA-P (parkinsonism), whilst if a cerebellar syndrome predominates, it is known as MSA-C.
- The abnormal protein found pathologically is alpha-synuclein.
- There is a poor response to levodopa.

Vascular Parkinsonism

- There is usually greater lower limb than upper limb involvement with (most commonly) slow progression of symptoms (rather than sudden onset).

Wilson's Disease

- This is an autosomal recessive disorder of copper metabolism (mutations in gene *ATP7B* on chromosome 13).
- A movement disorder is the most common neurological presentation. This can be an akinetic-rigid syndrome, tremor and/or dystonia.
- Neuropsychiatric features (behavioural change or depression) can also occur and occasionally there may be a cerebellar syndrome (particularly dysarthria).
- Non-neurological features include liver disease, Kayser–Fleischer rings and renal tubular acidosis.
- Investigations usually reveal a low serum copper, low serum caeruloplasmin and high urinary copper.
- Treatment is with pencillamine (first line), trientene or zinc salts.

Dyskinesias with Jerky Movements

Myoclonus

These are sudden, brief, jerky involuntary movements which can be generalised or focal.

Myoclonus can be physiological (e.g. hypnic jerks) but is often pathological and can occur as part of an epilepsy syndrome or in neurodegenerative diseases (e.g. CJD or CBD), in association with some cerebellar disorders (progressive myoclonic ataxia), due to metabolic disorders (e.g. in uraemia) or post-anoxia (Lance–Adams syndrome).

Chorea

These are excessive spontaneous involuntary movements that are irregular and jerky and may seem to flow from one part of the body to another.

Causes

- Genetic: Huntington's disease, neuroacanthocytosis, dentatorubro-pallidoluysian atrophy (DRPLA)
- Drugs: neuroleptics, levodopa, dopamine agonists, oral contra-ceptive pill
- Stroke (often causing hemiballism due to contralateral subthala-mic nucleus involvement)
- Other: chorea gravidarum, hyperthyroidism, antiphospholipid syndrome/SLE, polycythaemia vera, Sydenham's chorea

---

Huntington's Disease (HD)

- This is an autosomal dominant trinucleotide repeat disorder caused by mutations in the gene encoding the huntingtin protein on chromosome 4. It shows full penetrance and anticipation.
- The onset is usually between 30 and 50 years old, but it can present later or earlier.
- There is a triad of clinical features: motor (chorea and other movement disorders), cognitive (executive dysfunction initially) and psychiatric (depression, anxiety, irritability). Suicide is four times as common as the general population.
- Some patients present with an akinetic-rigid syndrome (Westphal variant), and this is more common in juvenile HD than in adult-onset disease.
- Genetic counselling is very important.
- If an MRI is performed, then bilateral caudate atrophy is seen.

Dyskinesias with Non-Jerky Movements

Tremor

A tremor is an involuntary, rhythmic alternating movement of one or more body parts. There are three main types.

Postural

- Physiological or exaggerated physiological, e.g. hyperthyroidism, alcohol withdrawal, sympathomimetic drugs.
- Essential tremor: may be familial, usually symmetrical, affecting the hands mainly, but also on occasion the head, voice and legs. It may be improved by alcohol but is worse with anxiety. It is treated with propranolol or primidone.

Rest

Characteristic of PD. Other akinetic-rigid syndromes often do not have a rest tremor although may have a postural tremor.

Kinetic (Intention)

This occurs during movement of a body part, e.g. cerebellar disease.

Dystonia

In dystonias, involuntary sustained muscle contraction leads to parts of the body being distorted into abnormal postures. Additional involuntary movements may occur. Dystonia may be primary or secondary to another disorder, e.g. stroke, and may be generalised or focal, e.g. torticollis (twisting of neck to one side) or blepharospasm (closure of the eyelid). It can also be task-specific, e.g. writer's cramp.

Rarely, it can present acutely e.g. oculogyric crisis (sustained upward deviation of the eyes often with accompanying involvement of the neck and mouth), commonly due to dopamine antagonists (metoclopramide, neuroleptics) and treated with anticholinergic drugs such as procyclidine.

Neuroleptic Malignant Syndrome

- Normally occurs within a few days of starting (or changing dose of) a neuroleptic (e.g. haloperidol, chlorpromazine, fluphenazine) and can occur after a single dose.

- Features include rigidity as well as fever, autonomic dysfunction (sweating, tachypnoea, tachycardia, labile blood pressure), confusion and altered consciousness, very high CK and a raised white cell count.
- Dantrolene and dopamine agonists are used (together with withdrawal of the offending drug).

Chapter 9

Multiple Sclerosis

Multiple sclerosis (MS) is an inflammatory, demyelinating disorder of the central nervous system (CNS).
Three main clinical subtypes are recognised:

- relapsing-remitting
- primary progressive
- secondary progressive (in those with previous relapsing-remitting)

Symptoms

Patients may present with an attack of focal neurological symptoms affecting any part of the central nervous system, but common presentations are:

- Spinal cord disease: spastic paraparesis, sensory impairment below the level of the lesion, bladder and/or bowel problems
- Optic neuritis: unilateral painful visual disturbance
- Brainstem/cerebellar disease: cerebellar syndrome, an internuclear ophthalmoplegia (which may be bilateral), other eye movement disorders, vertigo, facial weakness or numbness

To make a clinical diagnosis of MS, there must be evidence of at least two CNS lesions in different places at different times (dissemination in space and time), e.g. a single episode of optic neuritis does not fulfil criteria (it is a 'clinically isolated syndrome').

Two other clinical features which occur in demyelination are:

- Lhermitte's sign: a feeling of an electric shock running down the back and the legs on bending the neck forward
- Uhthoff's phenomenon: worsening or temporary reappearance of symptoms with heat, e.g. after a hot bath or exercise

Paroxysmal symptoms such as trigeminal neuralgia may occur occasionally. Patients may also develop fatigue, seizures and cognitive impairment as the disease develops.

Investigation

Investigations in someone presenting with possible MS include:

- Blood tests to exclude an autoimmune cause
- MR imaging of the brain and spine
- Lumbar puncture to look for the presence of unmatched oligoclonal bands in the CSF (indicating intrathecal IgG synthesis)
- Evoked potentials (e.g. visual)

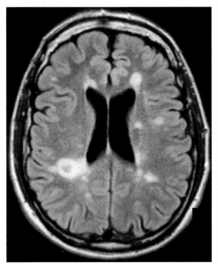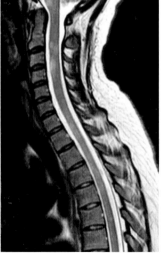

Fig. 5. MRI scans showing demyelination in the brain and spine.

Management

In acute relapses, high-dose steroids (either intravenously or orally) may be given to hasten recovery (although they do not affect the extent of recovery).

With increasing disease burden, a multi-disciplinary team approach becomes important with specialist nurse, physiotherapist and occupational therapist input. Symptomatic treatment of spasticity (e.g. baclofen or tizanidine) and bladder problems (e.g. oxybutynin) is often necessary. Amantadine or modafinil are sometimes given for fatigue.

Disease-modifying therapies include:

- beta-interferon
- glatiramer acetate
- mitoxantrone
- natalizumab (a monoclonal antibody against $\alpha 4$-integrin)

Chapter 10

Cerebellar Disease

Lesions of the cerebellar hemispheres tend to cause ipsilateral limb ataxia (dysmetria, intention tremor, dysdiadochokinesis, heel-shin ataxia), whilst lesions of the vermis cause gait and truncal ataxia. Other signs of cerebellar disease are eye movement disorders (particularly nystagmus, which may be maximal on looking towards the side of the lesion) and dysarthria (which has a slurred or staccato quality). Decreased tone in the limbs may be seen acutely.

Causes

The most common causes of cerebellar disease are:

- Multiple sclerosis
- Alcohol
- Space-occupying lesions, e.g. tumours
- Stroke

Other causes include:

- Paraneoplastic
- Infection/Inflammation: viral infection, e.g. Varicella–Zoster virus (VZV), Miller Fisher Syndrome
- Neurodegenerative: prion disease, multiple system atrophy
- Congenital: Arnold–Chiari malformation
- Hereditary: Friedreich's ataxia, spinocerebellar ataxias, ataxia telangiectasia, DRPLA, mitochondrial disease, Wilson's disease

- Endocrine/metabolic diseases: hypothyroidism, vitamin E or B12 deficiency
- Drugs/toxins: phenytoin, carbamazepine, lithium, amiodarone, ciclosporin

Friedreich's Ataxia

- Autosomal recessive trinucleotide repeat disorder (frataxin on chromosome 9).
- It usually starts before the age of 20.
- Cerebellar syndrome with spinal cord disease (corticospinal tract involvement leads to spastic paraparesis, dorsal column involvement leads to impaired proprioception and vibration sense) and peripheral nerve involvement (lower limb areflexia).
- Other features include scoliosis, pes cavus, deafness and cardiomyopathy.

Chapter 11

Cranial Nerve Disorders

The 12 cranial nerves can be affected by a number of different pathologies. A schematic way of thinking about this is by considering the path of each nerve in four parts: starting at the nuclei and then passing through the brainstem itself (1), then through the surrounding meninges (2), through the bony foramina in the skull (3), and finally finding its way on its pathway to the target (4). Common causes of cranial nerve palsies can then be thought of in these four places:

1. Brainstem

    - Space-occupying lesions
    - Stroke
    - Motor neurone disease
    - Multiple sclerosis
    - Encephalitis
    - Syringobulbia

In brainstem disease, cranial nerve palsies are ipsilateral, and there may be associated contralateral long tract signs (limb weakness or sensory impairment).

2. Meninges

    - Basal meningitis — TB, sarcoidosis, lymphomatous, carcinomatous
    - Meningioma

3. Bone

- Trauma
- Paget's disease

4. On its pathway to the target

- Cranial mononeuropathies: diabetes, inflammation (Miller Fisher syndrome, vasculitis), infection (herpes zoster, Lyme disease)
- Compressive pathologies: tumour, aneurysm, fistula, thrombosis
- Raised intracranial pressure

Some patients present with combinations of cranial nerve palsies which may be related to a mononeuritis multiplex, e.g. due to diabetes or vasculitis, or related to a specific anatomical syndrome:

- Superior orbital fissure/cavernous sinus syndromes: 3rd, 4th, 5th-ophthalmic division, 6th nerves
- Cerebellopontine angle lesions: 5th, 7th +/− 8th nerves
- Lateral medullary syndrome: 5th, 9th, 10th nerves
- Jugular foramen syndrome: 9th, 10th, 11th nerves

Palsies of the 2nd, 3rd, 4th and 6th Nerves

Optic nerve disease

This usually causes a decrease in visual acuity with loss of colour vision, a visual field defect and an afferent pupillary defect eventually leading to optic atrophy (pale optic disc on fundoscopy). Onset may be acute (e.g. optic neuritis or ischaemia), subacute (e.g. Leber's), or slowly progressive (e.g. toxins or vitamin deficiencies). Causes include:

- Inflammation (optic neuritis): MS, NMO, viral infections, SLE, syphilis
- Vascular: arteritic (i.e. giant cell arteritis) or nonarteritic ischaemic optic neuropathy
- Inherited: Leber's hereditary optic neuropathy

- Toxic/nutritional: methanol, vitamin B12 deficiency, tobacco/ alcohol amblyopia
- Drugs: ethambutol
- Compression: tumours

Visual Field Defects

In front of the optic chiasm

- Retinal disease: visual field loss depends on the part of the retina affected, e.g. peripheral in retinitis pigmentosa (leading to tunnel vision in advanced RP) or a central scotoma in macular disease.
- Optic nerve disease: usually results in a central scotoma (e.g. optic neuritis) but in anterior optic nerve disease there may be an altitudinal field defect (e.g. loss of the lower half of the visual field in ischaemic optic neuropathy).

At the optic chiasm

- Bitemporal hemianopia usually due to pituitary tumours

Behind the optic chiasm

Lesions cause a contralateral homonymous hemianopia (HH) or homonymous quadrantanopia (HQ):

- Optic tract: HH
- Upper optic radiation (parietal): inferior HQ
- Lower optic radiation (temporal): superior HQ
- Occipital cortex: HH (may be macular sparing, i.e. bilateral lesions may cause tunnel vision)

Pupil Abnormalties

Small pupil (Miosis)

The most common cause is Horner's syndrome. Other causes include pontine lesions, Argyll Robertson pupil, long-standing Adie's pupil and drugs (miotic eye drops, e.g. pilocarpine, opiates, organophosphate poisoning).

Horner's Syndrome

- This is due to a lesion of the sympathetic pathway. Causes can be split according to where in the pathway (consisting of three neurones) is affected:
- *Central* (i.e. from the hypothalamus through the brainstem to the spinal cord): stroke (lateral medullary syndrome), syringobulbia, tumours
- *Pre-ganglionic* (i.e. from the T1 root into the cervical sympathetic chain to the superior cervical ganglion): apical lung (Pancoast's) tumours, trauma to the neck, lymphadenopathy
- *Post-ganglionic* (i.e. after the ganglion, as it runs along the carotid artery to the eye): carotid dissection, cluster headache
- The triad of symptoms are miosis, partial ptosis and anhydrosis (loss of sweating on the affected side which may not occur in post-ganglionic lesions).

Argyll Robertson Pupil

- This is a small, irregular pupil with light-near dissociation, i.e. loss of reaction to light but intact reaction to accommodation. It is probably due to a midbrain lesion.
- Although classically seen in neurosyphilis, light-near dissociation is also seen in autonomic neuropathies (e.g. diabetes) and Parinaud's syndrome.

Large pupil (Mydriasis)

The most common cause is a third nerve palsy or an Adie's (myotonic) pupil (the Holmes–Adie syndrome includes absent deep tendon reflexes). Drugs can also cause a large pupil (mydriatic eye drops, e.g. tropicamide, tricyclic antidepressants, cocaine).

Relative afferent pupillary defect (RAPD or Marcus Gunn pupil)

This occurs with partial optic nerve lesions (e.g. in optic neuritis) and can be seen best with the swinging light test. The pupils appear equal initially. The light is shone in the unaffected eye causing constriction of both pupils as normally. However, when the light is swung to the affected eye, there is paradoxical dilation of the pupil. This is because there is a poor direct response to light in this eye (due to damage to the afferent pathway).

Eye Movement Disorders

Ophthalmoplegia can be thought of as being caused by a problem in one of five places: supranuclear (upper motor neurone), 3rd, 4th and 6th nerves (lower motor neurone), medial longitudinal fasciculus (interneurones), neuromuscular junction and muscles.

Supranuclear gaze palsies

These are caused by upper motor neurone problems (i.e. between the cortex and the brainstem nuclei) and can cause a complex ophthalmoplegia. Conditions in which they occur include:

- PSP where vertical gaze (down before up) is affected first.
- Parinaud's syndrome where upgaze is affected but downgaze is preserved. This is due to dorsal midbrain pathology, e.g. a stroke or tumours. Other eye abnormalities in this syndrome include convergence-retraction nystagmus and light-near dissociation of the pupils.

3rd, 4th, 6th nerve palsies

- Complete 3rd nerve palsies cause the eye to be held in a 'down and out' position with a complete ptosis and mydriasis. However, it may be partial and/or pupil-sparing. Compressive lesions (e.g. posterior communicating artery aneurysms) are often painful and

involve the pupil whilst non-compressive lesions (e.g. diabetes) are usually painless and may be pupil-sparing.
- 4th nerve palsies cause an inability to look downwards and inwards. Patients may tilt their head away from the side of the lesion.
- 6th nerve palsies cause a failure to abduct the eye.

Internuclear ophthalmoplegia

Internuclear ophthalmoplegia occurs when the interneurones between the 3rd and 6th cranial nerve nuclei within the medial longitudinal fasciculus (MLF) are affected. This can cause a failure of adduction on the side of the lesion with nystagmus in the contralateral eye (i.e. a right MLF lesion causes failure of adduction in the right eye and nystagmus in the left eye). It is most commonly caused by multiple sclerosis, where it is often bilateral.

Neuromuscular junction disorders

Problems in the neuromuscular junction can cause a complex ophthalmoplegia, i.e. myasthenia gravis.

Muscle disease

Problems in the muscles can cause a complex ophthalmoplegia:

- Thyroid eye disease (with proptosis and lid lag)
- Mitochondrial disease
- Muscular dystrophies, e.g. myotonic, oculopharyngeal

Palsies of the 5th Nerve

Isolated lesions of the 5th nerve are relatively uncommon but it can be affected as part of cavernous sinus syndromes, cerebellopontine angle lesions or brainstem disease, e.g. lateral medullary syndrome or multiple sclerosis.

Trigeminal Neuralgia

- Patients have intermittent episodes of sharp, stabbing pain lasting seconds that are most commonly in the distribution of the maxillary or mandibular branches of the trigeminal nerve.
- The pains may be triggered by eating or by touch.
- Examination is usually normal in between episodes with no facial sensation loss.
- MRI is necessary to exclude a compressive lesion or MS but many patients will have a normal scan and the presumptive cause is irritation from a small overlying blood vessel.
- Carbamazepine is the first-line treatment. Some patients eventually end up having surgical microdecompression.

Palsies of the 7th Nerve

Facial weakness may be caused by problems either in the corticobulbar tract (UMN, e.g. stroke, sparing the upper part of the face), the 7th nerve itself (LMN), the neuromuscular junction (myasthenia gravis) or muscle (e.g. myotonic dystrophy, facioscapulohumeral dystrophy).

7th nerve (LMN) palsy is most commonly a Bell's palsy (i.e. idiopathic) and may be preceded by pain behind the ear. Other causes include:

- Ramsay Hunt syndrome (due to herpes zoster and there may be associated vertigo, tinnitus and deafness. Vesicles may be seen in or around the ear.)
- Guillain–Barré syndrome (GBS)/Miller Fisher syndrome (MFS)
- Sarcoidosis
- Lyme disease
- Parotid gland tumours
- Middle ear infections
- Cerebellopontine angle tumours

If facial weakness is bilateral, it is most likely to be due to neuromuscular junction or muscle disease (particularly if symmetrical) but GBS/MFS, Lyme disease and sarcoidosis in particular can cause bilateral weakness.

Palsies of the 8th Nerve

The 8th nerve can be affected by many different pathologies causing one or more of deafness, tinnitus and vertigo.

Deafness

Hearing loss may be conductive (due to a problem between the outer and inner ear, e.g. middle ear infections, trauma, otosclerosis) or sensorineural (SNHL, due to a problem with the inner ear, cochlea or 8th nerve/nucleus). Causes of SNHL include presbyacusis and:

- Tumours: acoustic neuroma (vestibular schwannoma)
- Inherited: either as the only symptom, part of mitochondrial diseases or as part of a syndrome, e.g. Usher, Pendred, Alport syndromes
- Meniere's disease
- Vascular: brainstem infarction
- Autoimmune: SLE, polyarteritis nodosa (PAN), Cogan's syndrome
- Paget's disease
- Infection: zoster (Ramsay Hunt syndrome), TB
- Drugs: aminoglycosides, loop diuretics, quinine, NSAIDs

Vertigo

Patients presenting with a feeling of dizziness may not have true vertigo. Their symptoms may be caused by postural hypotension, arrhythmias, vasovagal syncope, anaemia or hypoglycaemia. Causes of true vertigo include:

- Benign paroxysmal positional vertigo
- Idiopathic vestibulopathy (vestibular neuronitis or labyrinthitis)

- Vascular: vertebrobasilar ischaemia/infarction
- Vestibular failure: ototoxic drugs, degenerative
- Others: multiple sclerosis, Meniere's disease, migraine

Benign Paroxysmal Positional Vertigo

- This is due to peripheral labyrinthine pathology and is usually idiopathic but may occur after an infection or trauma. There are sudden onset, brief episodes of vertigo (normally under 30 seconds) triggered by a change of position (e.g. lying down or turning to the affected side). Most patients are asymptomatic between episodes but occasionally some complain of an odd feeling for hours after.
- The Hallpike manoeuvre is diagnostic and management involves the Epley manoeuvre and/or vestibular rehabilitation exercises.

Palsies of the Lower Cranial Nerves (9th, 10th, 11th and 12th)

Bulbar palsy

This is caused by bilateral lower motor neurone lesions of the lower cranial nerves leading to nasal speech (bulbar or flaccid dysarthria) and dysphagia (particularly for fluids, with nasal regurgitation and coughing). On examination, there is weakness of the soft palate (difficulty saying 'aah') as well as wasting and fasciculations of the tongue. The gag reflex may be absent.

Causes include motor neurone disease and Guillain–Barré syndrome. Weakness of the bulbar muscles also occurs in myasthenia gravis and rarely in muscle disorders.

A pseudobulbar palsy is a disorder caused by bilateral upper motor neurone lesions, i.e. the corticobulbar tracts. Speech and swallowing are affected and speech may have a slow, indistinct and strangled quality (pseudobulbar or spastic dysarthria). The tongue is spastic and stiff so movements are slow. The jaw jerk is brisk. Patients often have labile affect (pathological laughter and crying).

Causes include motor neurone disease, cerebrovascular disease and MS.

Jugular foramen syndrome

This is the combination of 9th, 10th and 11th nerve palsies due to pathology as they pass together through the jugular foramen.

It is often due to compression from a tumour, including a rare vascular tumour known as glomus jugulare, which may also cause conductive hearing loss and pulsatile tinnitus.

Chapter 12

Disorders of the Spinal Cord

Spinal cord disease results in variable clinical features:

- Upper motor neurone signs below the level of the lesion +/– lower motor neurone signs at the level of the lesion
- Sensory impairment below the level of the lesion
- Bladder, bowel and sexual dysfunction

However, signs depend on how much of the cord has been affected:

1. Total cord syndrome

    - Spastic paraparesis or quadraparesis (in cervical lesions), although acutely there may be 'spinal shock' and features of a flaccid paraparesis
    - Impairment of sensation for all modalities below the level of the lesion (a 'sensory level')

2. Anterior cord syndrome, e.g. anterior spinal artery infarction

    - May have spastic paraparesis or quadraparesis
    - Pain and temperature impairment below level of lesion

3. Posterior cord syndrome, e.g. subacute combined degeneration

    - May have spastic paraparesis or quadraparesis
    - Vibration and proprioception impairment below level of lesion

4. Central cord syndrome, e.g. syringomyelia

    *   May have spastic paraparesis or quadraparesis
    *   Pain and temperature impairment over the levels of the lesion (for example C4 to C8)

5. Hemicord syndrome (Brown-Sequard syndrome)

    *   Ipsilateral hemiparesis (in high cord lesions affecting cervical cord) or monoparesis (in lower cord lesions, i.e. thoracic or lumbar cord)
    *   Ipsilateral vibration and proprioception impairment, as well as contralateral pain and temperature impairment

The schematic diagram in Fig. 6 explains the different cord syndromes:

*   The diagram represents a section through the spinal cord with the corticospinal tracts, dorsal columns and spinothalamic tracts shown. Also shown is a representation of the early decussation of spinothalamic tract fibres to the opposite side of the cord.

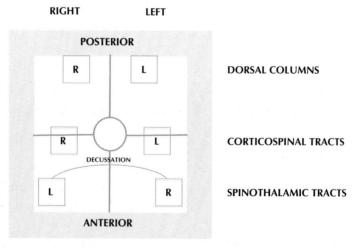

Fig. 6.   A schematic diagram explaining spinal cord syndromes.

- The letters R (for right) and L (for left) represent the side of the body affected by a lesion to a tract.
- Example 1: In a right hemicord syndrome there is right-sided pyramidal weakness (corticospinal tract), right-sided proprioception and vibration sense impairment below the level of the lesion (dorsal column) and left-sided pain and temperature sense impairment below the level of the lesion (spinothalamic tract).
- Example 2: In a central cord syndrome there is bilateral pain and temperature sense impairment over the affected levels (due to involvement of the decussating fibres of the spinothalamic tracts) and there may be bilateral pyramidal weakness (both corticospinal tracts).

Causes of spinal cord disease include:

- Degenerative: disc prolapse, spondylosis
- Inflammation: multiple sclerosis, transverse myelitis (can be post-infective), neuromyelitis optica, SLE, sarcoid
- Space-occupying lesions: tumours, abscesses
- Trauma
- Inherited: Hereditary spastic paraparesis, adrenoleukodystrophy
- Infection: TB, HTLV-1 (tropical), syphilis, Lyme disease, HIV
- Vascular: anterior spinal artery infarction, AVM
- Motor neurone disease
- Syringomyelia
- Subacute combined degeneration (B12 deficiency)

Disease above the brainstem can very rarely mimic spinal cord disease, e.g. bilateral hemispheric strokes or parasagittal meningioma.

Neuromyelitis Optica (NMO)

- Formerly known as Devic's disease, NMO is an autoimmune, inflammatory disorder associated with antibodies to aquaporin 4.
- Patients have a combination of an acute myelitis with an optic neuritis.

Hereditary Spastic Paraparesis (HSP)

- This is actually a heterogeneous group of disorders which can be 'pure' or 'complex', i.e. with other clinical features.
- Mutations in multiple genes have been described and inheritance may be autosomal dominant (e.g. due to spastin mutations), autosomal recessive (e.g. due to paraplegin mutations) or X-linked (e.g. due to PLP mutations).
- Pure HSP presents with progressive spasticity of the legs with brisk reflexes and extensor plantar responses (often with minimal weakness initially). Later on, there may be sensory disturbance, e.g. impaired vibration sense distally.
- In complex HSP other features may occur as well as the spastic paraparesis, e.g. optic atrophy, deafness, cerebellar features, akinetic-rigid features, sensory neuropathy.

Anterior Spinal Artery Infarction

- This causes an acute onset paraparesis which may be flaccid initially then spastic later on with impairment of pain and temperature below the level of lesion (with sparing of vibration and proprioception).
- There may be preceding sudden-onset, severe (radicular) back pain.

Syringomyelia

- Cystic cavitation in the spinal cord, often at a mid-cervical level.
- Clinical features are of a spastic paraparesis below the level of the syrinx, lower motor neurone signs at the level of the syrinx and loss of pain and temperature sensation (with sparing of vibration and proprioception) at the level of the syrinx. This may lead to a neuropathic arthropathy and/or trophic changes.

- The syrinx can expand into the brainstem and cause cranial nerve palsies.
- It may be associated with an Arnold–Chiari malformation and can be a late sequelae of trauma to the spine.

Investigations

Investigations for patients that present with a spastic paraparesis or quadraparesis include:

- Blood tests to look for inflammatory, infective or post-infective causes
- MR imaging of the spine (+/– brain)
- Lumbar puncture to look for evidence of inflammation (presence of white cells, increased protein and/or oligoclonal bands).

Chapter 13

Anterior Horn Cell Disorders

The anterior horn cell is affected in a number of different disorders:

- Motor neurone disease
- Infections: polio, West Nile virus
- Spinal muscular atrophy
- Spinobulbar muscular atrophy (Kennedy's disease)

Motor Neurone Disease (MND)

- This is a degenerative condition of the motor neurones causing motor signs with intact sensation (also known as amyotrophic lateral sclerosis, ALS). The mean age of onset is in the 60s.
- It is usually sporadic but about 5% of cases are genetic with mutations in multiple genes implicated (e.g. SOD1, TARDP, FUS).
- Neuropathologically, most cases of MND have abnormal TDP-43 deposition.
- Around a third of patients present with upper limb symptoms, a third with lower limb symptoms and a third with bulbar symptoms (speech and swallowing). A rare presentation is with respiratory muscle weakness. About 5% of patients develop frontotemporal dementia.
- In ALS, a mixture of upper and lower motor neurone features are seen. Onset can be with asymmetric findings in the

limbs or with bulbar symptoms, although patients eventually develop both limb and bulbar involvement.

- The other variants are much less common, e.g. lower motor neurone involvement only (progressive muscular atrophy) or upper motor neurone only (primary lateral sclerosis).
- It is a clinical diagnosis which can be supported by EMG.
- There is currently no curative treatment but the glutamate antagonist riluzole is usually given to patients as it may prolong the time before respiratory support is needed. Multidisciplinary team involvement is important.

Poliomyelitis

- Polio viruses are enteroviruses which are usually asymptomatic or cause a non-specific infection. However, in a very small number of cases they may cause a disorder of the anterior horn cells with asymmetrical (usually proximal greater than distal, legs greater than arms) weakness with lower motor neurone features, i.e. flaccidity, wasting and decreased/absent tendon reflexes.
- Despite a plan for worldwide eradication in forthcoming years via a vaccination programme, there are a number of areas in the world where polio remains endemic.

Chapter 14

Nerve Root and Plexus Disease

Radiculopathies

Nerve root disease may affect just one root (e.g. due to disc prolapse or compression from tumours or other space-occupying lesions) or many roots (e.g. inflammatory radiculopathies, multilevel disc disease, spinal stenosis). It often presents with neuropathic pain in the distribution of the nerve root although referred pain to other areas is common. The term sciatica is often used to describe pain and other symptoms due to lumbosacral nerve root disease.

Knowledge of anatomy is important to work out which nerve root is affected (see Chapter 1 on Basic Anatomy). However, a simple schematic is to ask yourself:

1. Which reflexes are affected? E.g. if the ankle jerk is affected then S1 is involved.
2. What is the pattern of sensory loss, i.e. which dermatome is involved?
3. Which movements are affected, i.e. which muscle groups are involved?

Cauda Equina Syndrome

This is a specific disorder of the collection of roots at the bottom of the spine known as the cauda equina. Causes include disc prolapse and space-occupying lesions. It is a neurosurgical emergency when due to an acute compressive lesion and patients need an urgent MRI scan and then referral for decompression if necessary. Clinical features are:

- Low back pain which may radiate to the legs
- A lower motor neurone syndrome of flaccid weakness and decreased or absent reflexes. The exact pattern depends on the level of the lesion and hence the roots affected.
- Saddle sensory abnormalities and poor anal sphincter tone are found on examination.
- Urinary retention or incontinence of urine and/or faeces due to bladder and bowel involvement.

Plexopathies

The brachial plexus is formed from the C5 to T1 roots. These form upper (C5, C6), middle (C7) and lower (C8, T1) trunks, which split into anterior and posterior divisions to form three cords: posterior (all three posterior divisions), lateral (anterior division of upper and middle) and medial (anterior division of lower). The radial and axillary nerves come off the posterior cord, the ulnar nerve comes from the medial cord and the median nerve comes from both the medial and lateral cords. The lumbosacral plexus is formed from the T12 to S5 roots with the lumbar plexus T12 to L5 and sacral plexus L4 to S5.

Common causes of plexopathies are trauma (including obstetric trauma), infiltration from carcinoma or lymphoma, inflammation, compression (e.g. from a cervical rib) and diabetes. Retroperitoneal disease, e.g. haematoma or fibrosis, can affect the lumbosacral plexus.

Brachial Neuritis (Neuralgic Amyotrophy)

- This is an inflammatory disorder of the brachial plexus that presents with severe pain around the shoulder and upper arm. This lasts for a few weeks with subsequent weakness (and sometimes wasting) of the shoulder girdle and upper arm muscles. There may be sensory loss over a patch on the upper arm. Most patients will improve over a few months but some have a longer recovery period and some are permanently disabled.

- It may occur sporadically but can follow trauma, surgery, infection or vaccination.

Traumatic Brachial Plexopathies

- **Erb's palsy** is a traumatic plexopathy of the upper part of the plexus (upper and middle trunks, i.e. C5, C6, C7 roots). Clinical features are variable but the arm is classically internally rotated with elbow extended and forearm pronated (the 'waiter's tip position').
- **Klumpke's palsy** is a traumatic plexopathy of the lower part of the plexus (lower trunk, i.e. C8, T1 roots). It causes weakness of the intrinsic muscles of the hand which may lead to clawing of the hand.

Diabetic Amyotrophy

- Although the exact site or cause of diabetic amyotrophy remains unclear, it most likely represents a lumbosacral plexopathy or radiculopathy.
- It is associated with type 2 diabetes and recent weight loss.
- Patients have unilateral (or more rarely, asymmetrical) proximal leg pain and weakness with later wasting. Knee reflexes are usually absent with intact ankle jerks. Sensory disturbance is usually absent or minimal although there may be an associated distal symmetrical sensory neuropathy.

Chapter 15

Mononeuropathies and Mononeuritis Multiplex

Mononeuropathies

Median neuropathy (Carpal tunnel syndrome)

This is very common and due to compression of the median nerve at the wrist. It is associated with arthritis, pregnancy, hypothyroidism, acromegaly and amyloidosis. Clinical features are:

- Pain and tingling in the fingers that may radiate up the arm and are worse at night but may be relieved by shaking the hand.
- There are often no abnormal signs but if severe there may be sensory disturbance in the median distribution (palmar thumb and 2½ fingers laterally) as well as wasting of the thenar eminence and weakness in muscles supplied by the median nerve (abductor and flexor pollicis brevis, opponens pollicis, lateral two lumbricals).
- Phalen's sign (sustained flexion of the wrist) and Tinel's sign (percussion over the carpal tunnel) may reproduce the symptoms but are not always positive and generally unreliable.

Nerve conduction studies are usually performed. Management is initially conservative with wrist splints but local steroid injection can be helpful and median nerve decompression may be necessary in some.

Ulnar neuropathy

This occurs usually at the elbow due to compression at the medial epicondyle and less commonly at the wrist. Clinical features are:

- Tingling and numbness in the little and ring fingers.
- There may be sensory disturbance in the ulnar distribution (1½ fingers medially) and wasting of the dorsal interossei and hypothenar eminence with weakness in the muscles supplied by the ulnar nerve (weak finger abduction and adduction and in severe cases there may be clawing of the hand).

Nerve conduction studies are usually performed. Management is conservative although surgery is occasionally performed.

Radial neuropathy

This is usually due to compression in the upper arm as the radial nerve passes around the humerus, classically in patients who are unconscious (or drunk — 'Saturday night palsy'). Clinical features are:

- Sensory disturbance on the dorsum of the hand (the 'anatomical snuffbox') and weakness of wrist and finger extension (wrist drop and finger drop).

Management is conservative with splints until it recovers (which occurs in most people). A lesion of the posterior interosseous branch of the radial nerve can also occur due to compression in the forearm. This causes finger drop but without wrist drop or sensory impairment.

Common peroneal neuropathy

This is often due to compression of the common peroneal nerve at the neck of the fibula, e.g. by a fracture or plaster cast, or by repeated crossing of the legs. Clinical features are:

- Variable sensory disturbance which may be only a small area over the dorsum of the foot in the web space between the big toe and adjacent toe (but in some cases can extend further onto the dorsum of the foot and the lateral aspect of the lower leg) and weakness of dorsiflexion (foot drop), eversion and big toe extension.

Management is conservative with a foot drop splint used until recovery.

Lateral femoral cutaneous neuropathy (meralgia paraesthetica)

This is due to compression as the nerve passes under the inguinal ligament causing tingling and numbness over an area on the lateral aspect of the thigh.

Femoral neuropathy

This nerve passes through the psoas muscle and can be affected by a psoas abscess or haematoma. Other causes include diabetes and trauma. Signs include weakness of knee extension, decreased or absent knee reflex and sensory disturbance affecting an area over the anteromedial part of the thigh.

Mononeuritis Multiplex

Patients may present with multiple mononeuropathies. The common causes of this are:

- Diabetes
- Vasculitis due to polyarteritis nodosa, Churg–Strauss syndrome, rheumatoid arthritis, SLE
- Sarcoidosis
- Lyme disease
- Amyloidosis
- Infiltration from lymphoma or carcinoma

Chapter 16

Peripheral Neuropathies

Polyneuropathies can be acute or chronic and present with weakness (usually distal and symmetrical) with lower motor neurone features and/or impairment of sensation, usually in a 'glove and stocking' distribution.

Acute Neuropathies

There are few disorders that cause an acute neuropathy: Guillain–Barré syndrome and its variants, vasculitis, porphyria, diphtheria and toxins/drugs.

Guillain–Barré Syndrome (GBS)

- This is an inflammatory radiculoneuropathy (i.e. root and nerve involvement) that is often post-infectious (*Campylobacter jejuni*, *Mycoplasma pneumoniae*, EBV, CMV)
- There is ascending symmetrical weakness (usually legs then arms) which reaches a peak within four weeks. Facial and bulbar muscles may become affected.
- Other features include sensory symptoms without signs, and autonomic dysfunction, i.e. arrhythmias, labile BP, urinary retention, constipation.

- Respiratory function needs to be monitored with regular vital capacity measurement and ICU involvement if it is decreasing.
- Lumbar puncture reveals a raised protein but normal white cell count. EMG shows a demyelinating picture in the classical acute inflammatory demyelinating polyneuropathy (AIDP) variant.
- IV immunoglobulins are first-line treatment. Patients require prophylactic anticoagulation and thromboembolic stockings to prevent deep vein thromboses.

Miller Fisher Syndrome

- This is a variant of GBS with the classic triad of ophthalmoplegia, ataxia (gait +/– limbs) and areflexia. Other features that may occur but are uncommon are mild limb weakness or sensory disturbance and facial weakness.
- Over 95% of patients will have antibodies to ganglioside GQ1b.

Porphyric Neuropathy

- This causes an acute motor axonal neuropathy and for this reason screening for porphyrins is usually undertaken in patients presenting with possible GBS.

Diphtheria

- Following a diphtheritic throat infection there is a biphasic course with an initial pharyngeal and palatal involvement leading to dysphonia and dysphagia followed by development of a demyelinating sensorimotor neuropathy affecting the limbs.

Chronic Neuropathies

Causes

The causes of chronic neuropathies can be classified according to the underlying pathology, i.e. whether they are axonal or demyelinating neuropathies (or both).

1. Axonal

   - Diabetes mellitus
   - Drugs: vincristine/other chemotherapy agents (e.g. cisplatin), isoniazid, nitrofurantoin/other antibiotics (e.g. metronidazole), ethambutol, gold, antiepileptic drugs (e.g. phenytoin), reverse transcriptase inhibitors
   - Deficiencies: vitamin B12, thiamine, pyridoxine
   - Alcohol
   - Autoimmune/vasculitis: Sjogren's syndrome, cryoglobulinaemia, RA, SLE
   - Metabolic/endocrine: uraemia, cirrhosis, hypothyroidism
   - Paraneoplastic
   - Some hereditary conditions (e.g. CMT2)
   - Infiltration: sarcoidosis, amyloidosis
   - Infection: HIV, leprosy, Lyme disease
   - Toxins: lead, arsenic, mercury

2. Demyelinating

   - Chronic inflammatory demyelinating polyneuropathy (CIDP)
   - Multifocal motor neuropathy (MMN)
   - Paraproteinaemic
   - Some drugs (e.g. tacrolimus, amiodarone)
   - Some hereditary conditions (e.g. CMT1, CMTX, Refsum's disease — an autosomal recessive disorder with excess phytanic acid)

Another way of classifying chronic neuropathies is according to whether they are pure or predominantly motor or sensory (or mixed sensorimotor):

- Motor: inflammatory neuropathies (e.g. CIDP, MMN), toxins (e.g. lead), drugs (e.g. dapsone)
- Sensory: diabetes mellitus, alcohol, Sjogren's syndrome, vasculitis, paraneoplastic

Palpable (thickened) peripheral nerves are seen in CMT disease, amyloidosis, neurofibromatosis, acromegaly and leprosy.

Investigations for neuropathies should include blood tests to look for causes mentioned above (FBC, urea and electrolytes, liver function tests, glucose, ESR, TFTs, ANA, ENA, ANCA, protein electrophoresis, B12/folate) as well as nerve conduction studies (which will tell you whether the neuropathy is axonal or demyelinating). Lumbar puncture may be performed if there is a possibility of an inflammatory neuropathy. If no diagnosis is made from these investigations then a nerve biopsy can be performed.

Charcot–Marie–Tooth (CMT) Disease

- This group of hereditary neuropathies has been variably classified over the years including the clinical terminology of hereditary motor and sensory neuropathy (HMSN). However, with increasing knowledge of the genetics of these conditions, a genetic classification is now preferred.
- CMT1 is the most common type (around 70% of cases) and is an autosomal dominant condition that starts towards the end of childhood. Mutations in the PMP22 gene are known to cause CMT1. Patients usually have a sensorimotor neuropathy with distal weakness and wasting in the legs and arms. Pes cavus and clawed toes may be present and peripheral nerves may be thickened.

- CMT2 is also autosomal dominant but less common than CMT1 with a slightly later onset and without the presence of thickened nerves.
- Other types are CMT4 which are the autosomal recessive cases and CMTX which are X-linked dominant cases.

Inflammatory Neuropathies

- CIDP is a chronic variant of GBS distinguished by the peak of the symptoms being longer than eight weeks. Like GBS it is an inflammatory radiculoneuropathy that may be predominantly motor but there is usually sensory involvement as well. It is either progressive or relapsing in nature. Nerve conduction studies show a demyelinating picture and CSF shows raised protein with a normal white cell count. IV immunoglobulins are often given although steroids can also be used.
- MMN is a rare progressive pure motor neuropathy causing asymmetrical upper greater than lower limb weakness. Fasciculations and wasting may be seen. Anti-GM1 ganglioside IgM antibodies are present in over half of patients.

Paraproteinaemic Neuropathies

- This is a group of disorders characterised by the presence of a paraprotein. Association may be with a monoclonal gammopathy of unknown significance or myeloma. One rare variant is POEMS: polyneuropathy, organomegaly, endocrinopathy, M-protein and skin changes.

Autonomic Neuropathies

- The autonomic nervous system may be affected in a number of different diseases including diabetes, amyloidosis and GBS.
- Symptoms include cardiovascular abnormalities (e.g. postural hypotension), erectile dysfunction, urinary symptoms (e.g. urgency, frequency), gastrointestinal symptoms (e.g. constipation, diarrhoea) and abnormal sweating.

Chapter 17

Neuromuscular Junction Disorders

Disorders of the neuromuscular junction include:

- Myasthenia gravis
- Lambert–Eaton myasthenic syndrome
- Botulism
- Congenital myasthenic syndromes

Myasthenia Gravis

- This is an autoimmune disease that causes weakness that is worse after prolonged muscle contraction (i.e. fatigability). It may be limited to the eyes (ocular myasthenia) or may be generalised.
- Patients commonly present with ptosis and ophthalmoplegia (diplopia) and, in generalised myasthenia, later develop limb, facial and bulbar weakness.
- In severe cases, a myasthenic crisis can occur with respiratory muscle weakness requiring ventilation — this may be triggered by intercurrent illness.
- EMG shows decrement on repetitive stimulation. Single fibre EMG shows jitter and block.
- Antibodies to the acetylcholine receptor (AChR) are found in 85% of generalised and 50% of ocular myasthenia. In those with generalised myasthenia who are negative for AChR antibodies, a proportion will have antibodies to muscle-specific kinase (MuSK).

- Edrophonium (Tensilon, a short-acting acetylcholinesterase inhibitor) may be given as a test dose to see if the weakness responds, but the test is only rarely performed.
- CT chest should be performed as 10–15% of patients have a thymoma.
- Symptomatic treatment is with the acetylcholinesterase inhibitor pyridostigmine. This can cause gastrointestinal problems (diarrhoea and abdominal cramps).
- In generalised myasthenia, immunosuppression is initially with prednisolone, with normally azathioprine as the first-line steroid-sparing agent.
- In acute exacerbations, intravenous immunoglobulins or plasma exchange can be used.
- Thymectomy is performed in young patients with generalised AChR antibody-positive disease.
- Some drugs can worsen myasthenia: aminoglycosides, ciprofloxacin, penicillamine, chloroquine.

Lambert–Eaton Myasthenic Syndrome

- This is an autoimmune disease associated with antibodies to voltage-gated calcium channels (VGCC).
- Around half of the cases are paraneoplastic with small cell lung cancer being the underlying disease in most patients.
- Patients have proximal limb weakness (in the lower limbs more than the upper limbs) with characteristic decreased or absent reflexes that return after a short period of sustained strong contraction of the relevant muscle group.
- Autonomic features are also seen (e.g. dry mouth, postural hypotension, GI and urinary problems).
- EMG shows reduction in the compound muscle action potential (CMAP) with increase following repetitive stimulation.

- Antibodies to VGCC are found in about 90% of patients.
- Treatment is of the underlying cancer if present and if no cancer is found screening should continue for at least five years.
- However, symptomatic treatment with the potassium channel blocker 3,4-diaminopyridine can be used.

Botulism

- This is caused by the anaerobic Gram-positive rod *Clostridium botulinum* and may be caused by food-borne disease or wound infection.
- Neurotoxins produced by the bacteria cleave presynaptic proteins preventing release of acetylcholine with resultant neuromuscular junction and autonomic nervous system dysfunction.
- There may be an initial period of gastrointestinal upset (nausea, vomiting, abdominal pain) prior to the onset of neurological symptoms.
- There is a descending flaccid paralysis with early symptoms of ophthalmoplegia, ptosis and bulbar weakness (dysarthria and dysphagia) followed by upper and then lower limb weakness. Reflexes remain intact and sensation is normal.
- These are followed by autonomic features: dilated, unreactive (or poorly reactive) pupils, dry mouth, postural hypotension, constipation and urinary retention.
- Samples of blood, stool and, if possible, the incriminating food sample should be sent to the local public health reference laboratory for detection of the toxin. EMG shows reduction in CMAPs.
- Supportive treatment is important and antitoxin may be given.

Congenital Myasthenic Syndromes

- These are rare and although they usually occur in infancy or childhood they very occasionally present in adulthood.
- They are mostly due to genetic mutations in proteins that are part of the neuromuscular junction (e.g. the acetylcholine receptor itself) and other proteins such as rapsyn and dok-7.
- They are not autoimmune diseases and do not respond to immunosuppression. Furthermore, pyridostigmine can cause deterioration in some of the syndromes.

Chapter 18

Muscle Disorders

Muscle disease usually presents with symmetrical proximal limb weakness and wasting. However, any other muscle group can be involved: face, eyes, bulbar, respiratory. Myalgia (muscle pain) or cramps occur in some conditions. Pseudohypertrophy is seen in Duchenne and Becker muscular dystrophy and some limb girdle dystrophies. Investigations for muscle disease should include creatine kinase (CK), electromyography (EMG) and, if the diagnosis is not clear, muscle biopsy may be performed.

Causes

Acquired

- Inflammatory: polymyositis, dermatomyositis, inclusion body myositis
- Endocrine: Cushing's syndrome, Addison's disease, thyrotoxicosis, hypothyroidism, acromegaly, vitamin D deficiency
- Drugs: alcohol, statins (usually myalgia rather than weakness), steroids

Inherited

- Muscular dystrophies: Duchenne, Becker, facioscapulohumeral, limb girdle, oculopharyngeal
- Myotonias: myotonic dystrophy, congenital myotonia
- Metabolic: glycogen storage disorders, fatty acid metabolism defects

- Mitochondrial: CPEO, Kearns–Sayre syndrome, MERRF, MELAS
- Channelopathies: periodic paralyses

Polymyositis/Dermatomyositis

- These are inflammatory myopathies that present with progressive symmetrical proximal limb weakness and, in some patients, myalgia. Dysphagia and neck weakness may be seen.
- They can occur on their own but may accompany other connective tissue diseases. There is an association with malignancy. Some patients develop interstitial lung disease.
- In dermatomyositis, a heliotrope rash over the eyelids, Gottron's papules (over the knuckles) and a red photosensitive rash may be seen.
- Treatment is with immunosuppression: steroids initially, then methotrexate or azathioprine.

Inclusion Body Myositis

- This is a progressive myopathy presenting usually from the 50s onwards and in men more commonly than women.
- Weakness may be more distal than proximal with involvement of the long finger flexors and foot dorsiflexors but quadriceps are often also involved.

Duchenne and Becker Muscular Dystrophy

- These are both caused by mutations in the gene coding for dystrophin on the X-chromosome (X-linked recessive inheritance). Mutations are often *de novo*.
- Progressive proximal limb weakness occurs. Other features include respiratory muscle involvement. Later, cognitive impairment and cardiomyopathy also occur.

- Patients with Duchenne muscular dystrophy are usually wheelchair-bound by their teens but Becker muscular dystrophy is milder and patients walk for longer.

Myotonic Dystrophy

- This is an autosomal dominant trinucleotide repeat disorder caused by mutations in the gene coding for myotonin protein kinase on chromosome 19 (in type 1). There is anticipation with a mean age of onset in the 20s or 30s.
- The characteristic feature is myotonia (e.g. difficulty opening hands or eyes quickly). This is worse in cold weather.
- Unlike most other muscle disorders, weakness is usually distally in the hands with bilateral ptosis, myopathic facial features, dysarthria and ophthalmoplegia also seen. Later, respiratory muscle involvement may occur.
- It is a multisystem disease whose features may be remembered with the ABCDE mnemonic: atrophy of the testes, balding (frontal), cataracts, cognitive impairment, cardiomyopathy, diabetes mellitus (more commonly, impaired glucose tolerance), ECG abnormalities (dysrhythmias, heart block), endocrine disease (goitre).
- There is a characteristic EMG of myotonic 'dive bomber' discharges.
- Management is mostly supportive with genetic counselling, annual review for multisystem features (ECG, glucose, eye exam for cataracts).

Mitochondrial Disorders

- These are usually maternally inherited via mitochondrial DNA.
- Chronic progressive external ophthalmoplegia (CPEO) causes an ophthalmoplegia with ptosis. A subset of CPEO is

the Kearns–Sayre syndrome in which there is early onset (under the age of 20) of ophthalmoplegia, ptosis, and retinitis pigmentosa as well as heart block, raised CSF protein and cerebellar ataxia.

- Myoclonic epilepsy with ragged red fibres (MERRF) is a disorder with seizures and cerebellar ataxia as well as proximal limb weakness.
- Myopathy, encephalopathy, lactic acidosis and stroke-like episodes (MELAS) is a disorder with the features in its title.

Chapter 19

Investigations

Neurogenetics

Trinucleotide repeat disorders

These are a group of genetic disorders caused by an expansion (increased number) of trinucleotide repeats in genes. They show anticipation, i.e. severity increases with each generation and there is an earlier onset. They can be split into those with a CAG repeat and those with other repeats.

1. CAG (codes for glutamine, Q, hence they are known as polyQ disorders)

   - Huntington's disease
   - DRPLA
   - SBMA (Kennedy's disease)
   - Spinocerebellar ataxias (some types, e.g. 1, 2, 3, 6, 7, 17)

2. Non-polyQ disorders (CGG, GAA, CTG, CAG)

   - Fragile X
   - Myotonic dystrophy
   - Friedreich's ataxia

Neurofibromatosis (NF)

This is two separate autosomal dominant conditions, NF1 and NF2.

- NF1 is due to mutations in the NF1 gene on chromosome 17 encoding neurofibromin. Diagnostic criteria require two or more of: >1 neurofibromas or one plexiform neuroma, axillary or inguinal freckling, >5 café-au-lait spots, Lisch nodules (iris hamartomas), optic gliomas, skeletal abnormalities, e.g. sphenoid dysplasia and a relative with NF1. Other features include other gliomas, renal artery stenosis, phaeochromocytomas and scoliosis.
- NF2 is due to mutations in the NF2 gene on chromosome 22 encoding merlin. Acoustic neuromas (which may be bilateral) are characteristic. Other brain or spinal cord tumours may occur, including meningiomas, gliomas and other schwannomas. Peripheral neurofibromas and cataracts also occur.

Tuberous sclerosis

This is an autosomal dominant condition presenting in childhood with seizures and learning difficulties. MRI brain findings include subependymal nodules which may be calcified. Other features include skin lesions (ash-leaf macules, shagreen patches, facial angiofibromas or adenoma sebaceum and periungual fibromas), retinal hamartomas as well as kidney, heart and lung involvement.

Neurometabolic disorders

Errors of inborn metabolism often have neurological features.

1. Lysosomal storage disorders

    - Niemann–Pick disease — this is a group of disorders (A, B and C). Type C is associated with a cerebellar syndrome, vertical supranuclear gaze palsy, dystonia and cognitive impairment as well as hepatosplenomegaly.
    - Gaucher's disease — deficiency of glucocerebrosidase leading to a number of clinical subtypes. In adults it may present with myoclonus, seizures and cognitive impairment associated with hepatosplenomegaly.

- Fabry's disease — deficiency of α-galactosidase which neurologically may lead to a painful neuropathy as well as an increased risk of stroke. Other features include renal failure, angiokeratomas and keratopathy.
- Metachromatic leukodystrophy — deficiency of arylsulfatase A which can present as cognitive impairment in adulthood.

2. Peroxisomal disorders

    - Adrenoleukodystrophy — an X-linked disorder. One form of this disorder, adrenomyeloneuropathy, may present in early adulthood with progressive spastic paraparesis, peripheral neuropathy and adrenal insufficiency. Raised plasma very long-chain fatty acids (VLCFA) levels are seen.

Other groups of neurometabolic disorders include amino acid and organic acid disorders (e.g. phenylketonuria), urea cycle disorders and disorders of fatty acid oxidation.

CSF Examination

Lumbar puncture allows examination of the cerebrospinal fluid. The most common indication is for the investigation of possible meningitis where particular features distinguish the different causes.

	White cells	Protein	Glucose	Other tests
Bacterial	N (L in partially treated disease)	++	<50% serum	Gram stain, culture
Viral	L	+	Usually normal	Viral PCR
TB	L (N early on)	+++	<50% serum	Ziehl–Neelsen stain, PCR and culture
Fungal	L	+++	<50% serum	India ink stain, cryptococcal antigen
Malignant	Usually L	++	Normal or low	Cytology

N = neutrophils, L = lymphocytes
Protein: + 0.4–1 g/dl, ++ 1–2 g/dl, +++ >2 g/dl

However, lumbar puncture is also performed in other conditions, particularly where inflammatory causes are in the differential diagnosis:

- Headache — in patients with suspected subarachnoid haemorrhage, CSF may be examined to look for the presence of xanthochromia.
- MS — lumbar puncture is often performed to look for the presence of intrathecal IgG synthesis, i.e. unmatched oligoclonal bands (present in CSF but not in a matched serum sample). This can also be positive in other conditions (although often those with a different clinical picture), e.g. vasculitis, sarcoidosis, SLE.
- Neuropathies — increased protein in GBS and CIDP.

Another reason to perform a lumbar puncture is to look at the opening pressure in patients with possible idiopathic intracranial hypertension.

Neurophysiology

Nerve conduction studies (NCS) and electromyography (EMG) are performed in the investigation of most peripheral nervous system and muscle disorders (from the anterior horn cell to the neuromuscular junction and muscle).

Neuropathies

For peripheral neuropathies, NCS help to separate patients into those with axonal and demyelinating neuropathies. A simple way of distinguishing them using motor NCS is by looking at the amplitude of the compound muscle action potential (CMAP) and the motor conduction velocity (although in practice other values may be necessary).

	Amplitude	Conduction velocity
Axonal	Reduced	Normal
Demyelinating	Normal	Reduced

Some small fibre neuropathies may have normal values with standard NCS but abnormal thermal threshold testing.

Neuromuscular junction disorders

In myasthenia gravis, EMG shows decrement on repetitive stimulation. Single fibre EMG can be useful in myasthenia showing the features of jitter and block.

In comparison to myasthenia, Lambert–Eaton myasthenic syndrome shows reduction in the CMAP with increase following repetitive stimulation.

Muscle disease

In primary muscle disease, small and short duration motor unit action potentials are seen.

In myotonic dystrophy there are characteristic myotonic 'dive bomber' discharges.

Brain Imaging

CT scanning is readily available and is therefore often used in emergencies, e.g. in patients presenting with acute headache who may have a subarachnoid or intracerebral haemorrhage, patients presenting with focal neurological signs who may have had a stroke and in patients with raised intracranial pressure who may have a space-occupying lesion. However, in many of these cases, it is only the availability and speed of CT that makes it likely to be the initial type of scan in preference to MRI. CT is sensitive for detecting acute haemorrhage and is superior to MRI when looking at disease related to the bone, e.g. base of skull. On a CT scan, acute blood or bone/calcification is white, CSF is black whilst old blood, ischaemia and oedema are various shades of grey (usually darker than brain tissue itself).

MRI scanning is useful for the investigation of many neurological disorders. Different types of MRI sequence are performed: T1 is useful for looking at anatomy, T2 and fluid attenuated inversion

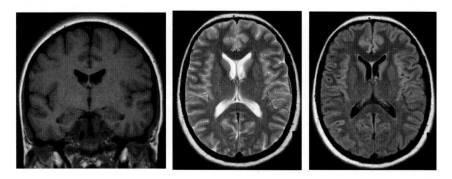

Fig. 7. *Examples of MRI scans showing coronal T1, axial T2 and axial FLAIR images.*

recovery (FLAIR) are useful for looking at white matter disease and diffusion weighted imaging (DWI) is most commonly used for investigating acute stroke. A simple way of identifying the different sequences is:

- T1: grey matter is grey, white matter is white, CSF is black
- T2: grey matter is white, white matter is grey, CSF is white
- FLAIR: as for T2 but CSF is black

Part 2

Neurological Examination for PACES

Chapter 20

Cranial Nerve Territory Examination

The Examination

- Observe the patient — particularly looking for ptosis, strabismus (squint or misalignment of the eyes) facial weakness and wasting
- Ask the patient if they have noticed any change in their sense of smell
- Eye examination

    1. Acuity

        a. Ask if they wear glasses normally
        b. You can say you would like to test acuity formally with a Snellen chart — this should be done with the patient's glasses on (if for distance vision) or, if these are unavailable, through a pinhole (improvement using the pinhole indicates a refractive error)

    2. Fields

        a. Ask the patient to describe any obvious field defect when looking at your face
        b. Peripheral — for each eye, bring in a moving finger from the periphery to the centre in all four quadrants (and *not* along the vertical and horizontal meridians)
        c. Central — for each eye, using a hat pin, find the blind spot then move the pin out of the blind spot up/down and left/right to map it out, comparing with your own blind spot

3. Pupils

    a. Observe size and shape
    b. Direct and consensual light reflex
    c. Accommodation reflex
    d. Swinging light test

4. Eye movements

    a. Pursuit movements looking for impaired movement and/or nystagmus
    b. Saccadic movements can be helpful, e.g. in an early INO

5. You can say that you would also test colour vision (with Ishihara plates) and perform fundoscopy

- Facial sensation and power

  1. Observe for facial asymmetry and wasting
  2. Sensation — test light touch with cotton wool in all three divisions of the 5th nerve, comparing both sides (and similarly, pain sensation with pinprick)
  3. Motor (5th) — opening mouth to resistance (jaw deviates to the side of the lesion), clenching teeth and feel the masseter and temporalis
  4. Motor (7th) — raise eyebrows, close eyes, blow out cheeks, show teeth
  5. You can say that you would also do the corneal reflex and perform the jaw jerk

- Hearing

  1. Whisper a number in the patient's ear with the opposite ear occluded
  2. If hearing is abnormal, then you should be prepared to perform (or say how you would perform) Rinne's and Weber's tests

- **Rinne's test**: using the 512 Hz tuning fork, test the difference between air conduction (AC — tuning fork next to the ear) and bone conduction (BC — tuning fork placed on mastoid). In a normal ear, AC is better than BC. In conductive hearing loss, BC is better than AC. In sensorineural hearing loss, the result is the same as the normal ear, i.e. AC is better than BC.
- **Weber's test**: using the 512 Hz tuning fork, place it in the middle of the forehead. In the normal patient, it should be heard equally in each ear. In conductive hearing loss, it is heard better in the affected ear whilst in sensorineural hearing loss it is heard better in the unaffected ear.

- Palatal movement

  1. Open mouth and say 'aah' — there should be symmetrical movement of the palate and uvula (which will move away from the side of any lesion)
  2. You can say you would check for a gag reflex as well as assessing speech and swallowing

- Trapezius and sternocleidomastoid power

  1. Shrug shoulders against resistance
  2. Turn head to each side against resistance whilst palpating the sternocleidomastoid to assess the bulk (opposite to the side the head is turned, i.e. the right sternocleidomastoid turns the head to left)

- Tongue movements

  1. Observe the tongue whilst it is in the mouth for any wasting, fasciculations or spasticity
  2. Ask the patient to stick their tongue out — it should protrude centrally (or towards the side of any lesion) and then check movements, particularly for their speed

Eyes

Summary of cases

- Ptosis
- Visual field defects

   a. Central visual field loss
   b. Peripheral visual field loss
   c. Bitemporal hemianopia
   d. Homonymous hemianopia
   e. Homonymous quadrantanopia

- Pupil abnormalities

   a. Large pupil (mydriasis)
   b. Small pupil (miosis)

- Eye movement abnormalities
- Nystagmus
- Cavernous sinus syndrome

Ptosis

Think about the pathway to the eyelid when considering the causes of ptosis (and be careful to look closely at the pupils):

- *3rd nerve*: 3rd nerve palsy — usually unilateral and may be a complete ptosis if there is a total 3rd nerve palsy but 3rd nerve palsies are often partial so the ptosis may also be partial. Usually an associated ophthalmoplegia +/− large pupil.
- *Sympathetic pathway*: Horner's syndrome — usually unilateral and ptosis is partial. There will be an associated small pupil.
- *Neuromuscular junction*: myasthenia gravis — may be bilateral and usually fatigable. It may be associated with complex ophthalmoplegia.
- *Muscle*: myotonic dystrophy, other muscular dystrophies (e.g. oculopharyngeal muscular dystrophy), mitochondrial

myopathies — usually bilateral, wasting may be present and there may be an associated ophthalmoplegia.

Visual field defects

The most common field defects seen are:

- Central field loss (scotoma) — usually due to optic nerve disease (see Part 1 for a list of causes) but may be due to macular disease.
- Concentric peripheral field loss (tunnel vision) — usually due to retinal disease, e.g. retinitis pigmentosa, some optic nerve diseases, e.g. chronic papilloedema, glaucoma and rarely bilateral occipital lobe disease (e.g. bilateral PCA infarcts).
- Bitemporal hemianopia — due to disease at the optic chiasm, e.g. a pituitary tumour. (Note that this may present initially as an upper bitemporal quadrantanopia because the inferior fibres of the chiasm are compressed first.)

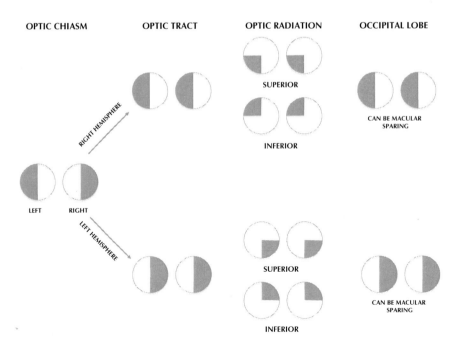

Fig. 8.   A diagram showing visual field defects.

- Homonymous hemianopia — usually due to occipital lobe disease (commonly a posterior cerebral artery infarct) rather than optic tract disease. Issues of macular sparing or incongruity are rarely important in the exam. (More anterior lesions may be incongruous but this is not reliable.)
- Homonymous quadrantanopia — the superior optic radiation (in the parietal lobe) represents the lower field on the contralateral side and the inferior optic radiation (in the temporal lobe) represents the upper field on the contralateral side.

Pupil abnormalities

Anisocoria is the term for unequal pupil size — around 20% of people will have a simple anisocoria, i.e. only 1 mm difference in size with intact pupillary reflexes.

- Small pupil (miosis) — the most common cause is Horner's syndrome (make sure you have not missed a subtle partial ptosis). The anisocoria will be maximal in dim light. Remember that the Argyll Robertson pupil is small (although usually irregular) and pontine lesions, e.g. haemorrhages, may cause miosis.
- Large pupil (mydriasis) — there are not many causes and assuming no systemic or topical drug use then this is likely to be due to a 3rd nerve palsy (look for associated ophthalmoplegia and ptosis) or an Adie's (myotonic) pupil (look for absent deep tendon reflexes — the Holmes–Adie syndrome).

Eye movement abnormalities

There are three main points to consider when examining an abnormality of eye movements:

1. *Is it a single nerve palsy?* These are usually unilateral. A 6th nerve palsy, i.e. failure of abduction, is the easiest to work out. Similarly, the additional features of ptosis +/– a large pupil in combination with impaired eye movements (adduction and/or vertical movements) point to involvement of the 3rd nerve. In a complete 3rd

nerve palsy, the eye will be down and out with a complete ptosis +/–
a large pupil. However, 3rd nerve palsies are often partial and these
findings may be variable. It is rare for a 4th nerve palsy, i.e. difficulty looking downwards and inwards, to be an isolated finding.

2. *If not a single nerve palsy, is it an internuclear ophthalmoplegia
   (INO)?* This may be unilateral but is often bilateral. This is failure of adduction (on the side of the lesion) which may be
   associated with nystagmus in the contralateral abducting eye.

3. *If not a single nerve palsy or INO, then it is essentially a 'complex ophthalmoplegia'.* This may be due to a combination of
   single nerve palsies, e.g. in Miller Fisher syndrome, a cavernous
   sinus syndrome or other multiple cranial nerve palsies. Thinking
   about the pathway that leads from cortex to muscle, eye movement abnormalities that are not due to cranial nerve
   abnormalities must be due to problems either below (neuromuscular junction and muscle) or above (upper motor neurone) the
   cranial nerves, i.e. the causes of a 'complex ophthalmoplegia' are:

   - Myasthenia gravis
   - Thyroid eye disease (which is a disease of the muscles)
   - Other muscle diseases, e.g. mitochondrial disorders or mus-
     cular dystrophies
   - Supranuclear gaze palsies (describes any UMN gaze palsy and
     due to multiple causes including trauma, tumours, stroke and
     degenerative disorders such as PSP) — these are relatively rare
     in the MRCP exams (and more strictly are gaze palsies, e.g.
     vertical or horizontal, rather than 'complex ophthalmople-
     gias'). The vestibulo-ocular reflex (tested with the 'doll's head
     manoeuvre') is intact in supranuclear palsies.

   If you find a 'complex ophthalmoplegia', think about whether
there are other findings pointing to one of these causes, e.g myopathic facial features, exophthalmos, fatigable ptosis.

Nystagmus

Nystagmus can be considered as being due to either a 'peripheral' or
'central' (i.e. cerebellar or brainstem) cause. Nystagmus has a slow

phase (drift away from the point of fixation) and a fast phase (a correction towards the point of fixation). The direction of nystagmus is defined by the fast phase and is towards the side of the lesion in 'central' causes and away from the side of the lesion in 'peripheral' causes. In reality, this is rarely important in the MRCP exam where the cause is usually central, e.g. you may be asked to examine eye movements and all you find is horizontal nystagmus — you may then be asked to examine further to see if there are other cerebellar findings.

Vertical nystagmus is caused by central lesions: downbeat nystagmus is classically associated with foramen magnum lesions, e.g. Arnold–Chiari malformations, but can also occur in cerebellar lesions.

Cavernous sinus syndrome

This is the association of 3rd, 4th and 6th nerve palsies with involvement of the 1st (and sometimes 2nd) division of the 5th nerve. There are a number of causes including cavernous sinus thrombosis, carotico-cavernous fistula, aneurysms, tumours (e.g. meningioma, pituitary adenoma) and inflammation (Tolosa-Hunt syndrome). There may be associated proptosis and chemosis in some cases. A similar combination of cranial nerve palsies is seen in lesions around the superior orbital fissure.

Face

> #### *Summary of cases*
>
> - Facial weakness — upper motor neurone, lower motor neurone, neuromuscular junction or muscle disorders
> - Cerebellopontine angle lesions

Facial weakness

Facial weakness can occur because of a disorder at the level of the upper motor neurone, lower motor neurone, neuromuscular junction or muscle. UMN and LMN lesions are usually unilateral (and distinguished by sparing of the forehead in UMN lesions) whilst NMJ and muscle disorders usually cause bilateral weakness.

Causes include:

- UMN — usually a stroke
- LMN — most commonly Bell's palsy, an idiopathic 7th nerve palsy. Other causes are listed in Part 1. Bilateral 7th nerve lesions occur in GBS/MFS, Lyme disease and sarcoidosis.
- NMJ — myasthenia gravis
- Muscle — causes include myotonic dystrophy and facioscapulo-humeral dystrophy

Cerebellopontine angle lesions

The most common cause is an acoustic neuroma (vestibular schwannoma) although other masses (e.g. meningiomas) may also cause the same syndrome. There is a combination of absent corneal reflex (which may be an early sign), abnormal facial sensation (5th nerve palsy) and facial weakness (7th nerve palsy). Acoustic neuromas affect the 8th nerve and cause sensorineural hearing impairment. In the exam you might notice that the patient has had the tumour removed and that a surgical scar is visible behind the ear.

Lower Cranial Nerve Territory

Summary of cases

- Bulbar and pseudobulbar palsies
- Lateral medullary syndrome
- Jugular foramen syndrome

Bulbar and pseudobulbar palsies

The bulb is the medulla and therefore a bulbar palsy is one involving the cranial nerves in the medulla (bilateral LMN lesions) so the patient is dysarthric (nasal speech or bulbar/flaccid dysarthria) and has a weak cough with weakness of the soft palate (difficulty saying 'aah'), a decreased or absent gag reflex and a wasted, fasciculating tongue on examination. Causes include motor neurone disease and Guillain–Barré syndrome. Myasthenia gravis may affect bulbar muscles as well.

A pseudobulbar palsy is caused by bilateral upper motor neurone lesions in the pathway to the bulbar nuclei, i.e. the corticobulbar tracts. There may be a spastic/pseudobulbar dysarthria (slow, indistinct and strangled) and, on examination, there is a brisk jaw jerk with a stiff spastic tongue (slow tongue movements). Causes include motor neurone disease, cerebrovascular disease and MS.

Lateral medullary syndrome

This is due to infarction of the posterior inferior cerebellar artery and, on examination, causes:

- Ipsilateral Horner's syndrome
- Ipsilateral pain and temperature sensory disturbance in the face
- Dysarthria
- Ipsilateral cerebellar signs
- Contralateral pain and temperature sensory disturbance in the limbs

Jugular foramen syndrome

This is a combination of 9th, 10th and 11th nerve palsies causing:

- Sensory disturbance of the soft palate ipsilaterally
- Decreased or absent gag reflex and hoarse voice
- Weakness of the ipsilateral sternocleidomastoid and trapezius

Speech

Summary of cases

- Dysarthria
- Dysphasia

Dysphonia is difficulty with phonation, i.e. with the vocal cord apparatus leading to an abnormality of the voice which may sound hoarse, weak or breathy. It would be very unusual to be asked to examine anyone with a dysphonia and, in general, speech examination is rare in the MRCP exam. However, if you are asked to examine speech, it is likely that the problem will be one of dysarthria, i.e. a problem with articulation, or dysphasia, a problem with language.

Examination of a patient with speech problems

Listen to spontaneous speech — it is important to get the patient to talk for a short period (around 30 seconds) to get an impression of their speech. The key question is whether they have a dysarthria, dysphasia or both. Asking questions like 'How did you get here today?' or 'What did you have for breakfast?' are likely to be unhelpful as they may generate single word answers. Asking the patient to describe a picture or to describe the room may be more helpful in generating a short passage of speech.

The key things to think about when listening to the speech are:

- *articulation* — are they having difficulty articulating the words?
- *fluency* — are they fluent or non-fluent?
- *grammar* — are they agrammatic ('telegraphic' speech)?
- *paraphasias and neologisms*– are there errors or made-up words in the speech?

If there are articulatory problems and this is a dysarthria, you can go on to try to distinguish between the dysarthrias:

- *repetition of simple sounds* — /pa/, /ta/ and /ka/
- *repetition of complex phrases* ('West Register Street', 'British Constitution', 'baby hippopotamus') — these are difficult for patients with any dysarthria and in patients with a cerebellar disorder they will be broken up into individual 'staccato' phrases

If there are no articulatory problems and this is a dysphasia, then you can go on to try to distinguish between the dysphasias:

- *comprehension* — 1-, 2- and 3-stage commands
- *naming* — high and low frequency words (e.g. watch, strap, buckle)
- *repetition* — polysyllabic words (e.g. city, citizen, citizenship)

Dysarthria

- Bulbar (flaccid) dysarthria — speech is nasal in quality
- Pseudobulbar (spastic) dysarthria — speech is slow, indistinct and strained or strangled
- Cerebellar dysarthria — speech is slurred or 'staccato'

The hypokinetic dysarthria of Parkinson's disease, i.e. soft, slow monotonous speech is usually easily distinguished as is the hyperkinetic dysarthria seen with dyskinesias.

Dysphasia

The main cause of dysphasia is stroke but any pathology affecting the perisylvian language areas in the dominant hemisphere can cause language impairment (e.g. tumours, neurodegenerative conditions such as Alzheimer's disease or frontotemporal dementia). In reality the anatomy of language is much more complicated than Broca's and Wernicke's areas but these still dominate most general physician's (and some neurologist's) thoughts on language.

	Broca's aphasia	Wernicke's aphasia
Fluency	Non-fluent (often to the extent it may sound dysarthric)	Fluent
Grammar	Speech may be 'telegraphic'	Normal
Paraphasias/neologisms	Sound errors (phonemic paraphasias)	Meaning errors (semantic paraphasias) and neologisms (jargon) more than sound errors
Comprehension (single word)	Normal	Impaired
Naming	Abnormal	Abnormal
Repetition	Impaired	Impaired

In conduction aphasia speech is fluent but there are problems with repetition in particular. Other stroke aphasias that have been described are the transcortical aphasias, transcortical motor aphasia and transcortical sensory aphasia, which are similar to Broca's and Wernicke's aphasia but have intact repetition.

Chapter 21

Limb Examination

The Examination

- Observation

  1. Wasting — be careful to look at the shoulder girdle and the small muscles of the hand, which are often overlooked.
  2. Fasciculations — these are best elicited by careful observation of muscles for around 30 seconds, paying particular attention to the deltoids, quadriceps and calf muscles.
  3. Abnormal movements — with the arms both at rest and outstretched, observe for the presence of a tremor.
  4. Biopsy scars — nerve biopsies are most commonly taken from the sural nerve behind the lateral malleolus whilst muscle biopsies may be taken from a variety of sites.

- Tone

  1. This should be examined in the upper and lower limbs. Clonus should be tested for in the lower limbs (ankles).
  2. Increased tone may be due to spasticity (an upper motor neurone lesion) or lead-pipe (with or without cogwheel effect due to superimposed tremor) rigidity (seen in parkinsonism).

- Power

  1. Test one muscle group at a time, comparing both sides and making sure to support above the joint you are testing.
  2. In the upper limb, shoulder abduction, elbow flexion and extension, wrist flexion and extension, finger flexion and extension, finger abduction (little finger and index finger

separately) and thumb abduction should be done as a minimum.

3. In the lower limb, hip flexion and extension, knee flexion and extension, ankle dorsiflexion and plantarflexion and big toe extension should be done as a minimum.

4. The muscles, nerves and nerve roots involved in these movements are shown in Part 1.

- Reflexes

    1. In the upper limb, biceps (C5,6), triceps (C7,8) and supinator (C5,6) reflexes should be tested.

    2. In the lower limb, knee (L3,4), ankle (S1,2) and plantar reflexes should be tested. With the plantar reflex, the big toe should move downwards normally, but in upper motor neurone lesions there will be a Babinski sign, i.e. the big toe will move upwards and the other toes fan out.

    3. If the reflexes cannot be elicited initially, then try with reinforcement — ask the patient to clench their teeth or hands.

    4. Hyperreflexia is seen in upper motor neurone lesions. There may be spread of reflexes to other muscle groups, e.g. crossed adductor reflexes (L2-4). Other findings include a positive Hoffman's sign and brisk finger jerks (C8).

    5. An 'inverted' reflex is when the movement elicited is different to the one normally seen (strictly, it should be opposite), e.g. in an inverted supinator jerk, finger flexion is seen instead of elbow flexion. This is due to a combined spinal cord and root lesion (e.g. cervical disc disease), affecting the root (LMN) at the level of the lesion (in this case C5/C6) causing an absent normal reflex, but also affecting the corticospinal tract (UMN) below the level of the lesion, causing hyperreflexia below (in this case C8 eliciting a finger jerk).

- Coordination
    1. In the upper limb, finger-nose testing and alternating hand movements should be performed.
    2. In the lower limb, heel-shin testing should be performed.

- Sensation — examination is carried out distally to proximally, comparing the two sides. Keep in mind what you have already found in the motor exam, e.g. in a patient with distal symmetrical weakness, you may find distal sensory loss, and in a patient with asymmetrical LMN weakness, you may find a dermatomal or single nerve pattern of loss.

  1. Start with light touch using a piece of cotton wool. Touch the sternum to give the patient a reference, then touch the patient's limb asking the patient two questions: can they feel it and does it feel the same as on the sternum?
  2. Pain sensation is tested with a pin ('Neurotip') using the sharp part in the same manner as with the cotton wool.
  3. Vibration sense is tested using a 128 Hz tuning fork, again using the sternum as a reference then starting distally and moving proximally in each limb until it is felt as normal.
  4. Proprioception is tested by moving the end of the finger at the distal interphalangeal joint or the end of the big toe at the interphalangeal joint, and asking the patient if they can sense whether it is being moved up or down. If they are unable to sense this, move proximally until the patient can perceive it normally.

- The lower limb examination should be completed by observing gait and performing Romberg's test. Some people like to observe gait at the start of a lower limb examination with the benefit of knowing what it shows going into the rest of the examination. However, gait assessment can be difficult and many signs pointing to the correct diagnosis will be seen in the rest of the limb examination. The key abnormal gaits to observe are:

  1. Parkinsonian gait
  2. Ataxic gait
  3. Spastic gait
  4. Waddling gait
  5. High-stepping gait
  6. Hemiplegic gait

The key to the limb examination in neurology is recognising patterns:

- **Parkinsonism** — these patients have features of bradykinesia, rigidity and a tremor but do not have weakness. In the exam, the clue to the patient having parkinsonism may be observation of their gait or of the presence of a tremor.

Examination of a patient with parkinsonism

- Observation for rest tremor, hypomimia ('masked face'), decreased blink rate. You may be asked to watch the patient walk initially and there will be difficulty with initiation, stooped posture, slow, shuffling movements with decreased arm swing and difficulty turning.

Initially look for the triad of features of tremor, bradykinesia and rigidity:

- Is there a rest tremor? Get the patient to put their hands on their knees and observe. This can be brought out by distraction.
- Is there a postural tremor? Get the patient to put their arms outstretched in front of them.
- Is there bradykinesia? Ask the patient to perform fine finger movements.
- Is there 'lead-pipe' or cogwheel rigidity? Examine the tone in the upper limb. This can be brought out by synkinesis (asking the patient to move their other arm).

Other parkinsonian features that might be elicited are micrographia (asking the patient to write a sentence), the hypokinetic dysarthria (asking the patient to speak) or the gait if you have not already done this.

The rest of the exam can be used to look for other causes of parkinsonian syndromes:

- Eye movements — is there a vertical gaze palsy as seen in PSP?
- Cerebellar exam — are there cerebellar features as seen in MSA?
- Lying and standing blood pressure — is there postural hypotension as seen in MSA?
- MMSE — is there cognitive impairment as seen particularly with DLB?

You may ask to do these things rather than actually incorporate them into the exam and you may also want to ask about a drug history (antipsychotic use in drug-induced parkinsonism).

- **Cerebellar syndromes** — these patients have coordination problems but do not have weakness. In the exam, the clue to the patient having a cerebellar syndrome may be observation of their ataxic gait or the presence of nystagmus on examination of eye movements.

Examination of a patient with a cerebellar syndrome

- Eye movements, looking for nystagmus.
- Speech (repetition of 'British Constitution', 'West Register Street', 'baby hippopotamus'), looking for slurred or staccato speech.
- Finger-nose testing, looking for past-pointing/dysmetria and an intention tremor.
- Alternating hand movements, looking for dysdiadochokinesis.
- Heel-shin testing, looking for lower-limb incoordination.
- Gait, looking for the broad based unsteady ataxic gait.

- **Impaired sensation** — remember that the spinothalamic tracts (which are anterior in the cord) carry pain (pin prick) and temperature (not usually tested in the MRCP exam) and the dorsal columns (which are posterior in the cord) carry proprioception and vibration sense whilst both tracts carry light touch. Patterns of sensory loss are:

  1. Distal symmetrical loss ('glove and stocking') — seen in peripheral neuropathies
  2. Loss in a single nerve distribution — seen in a mononeuropathy
  3. Loss in a dermatomal pattern — seen in root and plexus disease
  4. Loss below a sensory level — seen in spinal cord disease
  5. Hemisensory loss — seen in brainstem, thalamic, internal capsule and cortical disease

- **Weakness** — this is due to impairment in the motor pathway and is at one of four levels:

  1. Upper motor neurone (UMN): weakness is in a pyramidal pattern (i.e. weaker extensors in the upper limb and weaker flexors in the lower limb) and may be a paraparesis or quadraparesis with spinal cord disease, monoparesis if a lower hemicord disease (Brown-Sequard) or hemiparesis with upper hemicord, brainstem, internal capsule or cortical disease. There is accompanying spasticity, clonus, brisk reflexes and upgoing plantars.
  2. Lower motor neurone (LMN): the pattern of weakness is variable (e.g. distal and symmetrical in peripheral neuropathies, or unilateral/asymmetrical in mononeuropathies, root and plexus disease) but there may also be additional features of wasting, fasciculations, normal or decreased tone and decreased or absent reflexes.
  3. Neuromuscular junction (NMJ): weakness may be proximal and symmetrical and usually fatigable.
  4. Muscle: weakness is usually proximal and symmetrical and there may be wasting with normal or decreased reflexes.

	Inspection	Tone	Power	Reflexes
UMN	Usually normal — if severe, limb may be held in abnormal position	Increased (spasticity)	Pyramidal weakness — hemiparesis, monoparesis, paraparesis or quadraparesis	Increased with spread of reflexes and extensor plantars
LMN	Wasting Fasciculations	Normal or decreased (flaccidity)	Unilateral or asymmetrical limb weakness or distal symmetrical weakness	Decreased or absent
NMJ	Normal — may be associated ptosis and ophthalmoplegia	Normal	Usually proximal symmetrical weakness that is fatigable	Normal
Muscle	Wasting — may be associated myopathic facial features	Normal	Usually proximal symmetrical weakness	Normal or decreased in long-standing disease

Movement Disorders

Summary of cases

- Parkinsonism
- Hyperkinetic movement disorders, e.g. chorea

Parkinsonism

The examination of a patient with a parkinsonism is described above and the differential diagnosis is described in Chapter 8 of Part 1. The most common cause by far is idiopathic Parkinson's disease where there is asymmetrical rest tremor, bradykinesia and rigidity. Symmetrical rigidity early on is suggestive of another parkinsonian syndrome rather than PD. The other akinetic-rigid syndromes tend to have a postural tremor and not a rest tremor.

Hyperkinetic movement disorders

It would be rare to be asked to examine a patient with a hyperkinetic movement disorder in the MRCP exam but patients with parkinsonism may also have dyskinesias due to levodopa therapy. The differential diagnosis of chorea is described in Chapter 8 of Part 1.

Cerebellar Disorders

Summary of cases

- Cerebellar syndrome

Cerebellar syndrome

The examination of a patient with a cerebellar syndrome is described above and the differential diagnosis is described in Chapter 10 of Part 1. Remember that lesions cause ipsilateral signs and also that some causes are likely to result in unilateral disease (stroke, tumours) whilst others will cause bilateral signs (alcohol, hereditary ataxias, neurodegenerative disease).

Signs outside the cerebellum may help to make the diagnosis, e.g. spastic paraparesis and INO in MS, or spastic paraparesis, dorsal column involvement and lower limb areflexia in Friedreich's ataxia.

Pure Sensory Disorders

Summary of cases

- Sensory neuropathy

Sensory neuropathy

Some patients in the MRCP exam will have a normal motor examination but are then found to have a 'glove and stocking' sensory neuropathy. The causes of this are described in Chapter 16 in Part 1.

Upper Motor Neurone Disorders

Summary of cases

- Spastic paraparesis/quadraparesis
- Spastic hemiparesis
- Spastic monoparesis, including Brown-Sequard syndrome

Spastic paraparesis/quadraparesis

This is the most common of the upper motor neurone disorders seen in the MRCP exam. It is likely you will be asked to examine only the upper or lower limbs. If you only examine the lower limbs, you may find a paraparesis and be unaware whether the upper limbs are also affected — be sure to mention this at the end of the examination.

If you are allowed to perform a sensory examination, it is likely there is a sensory level. Review Chapter 12 for the different cord syndromes: total cord (all the sensory modalities), anterior cord (pain and temperature affected only, e.g. anterior spinal artery infarction), posterior cord (vibration and proprioception affected only, e.g. subacute combined degeneration of the cord) and central cord syndromes (spinothalamic tract sensory loss over the levels affected but not below the level, e.g. syringomyelia).

The differential diagnosis of spastic paraparesis/quadraparesis is also given in Chapter 12 as well.

There may be clues to the diagnosis in the examination, e.g. it is traditional in the MRCP exam to examine the back for surgical scars if you have found a spastic paraparesis or quadraparesis, which may indicate surgery for a space-occupying lesion or disc prolapse. In MS, there may be signs of other central nervous system involvement, e.g. cerebellar signs or INO. The sensory findings may also help (see above). In hereditary spastic paraparesis, there may be spasticity with minimal weakness.

Spastic hemiparesis

Hemiparesis is a common neurological disorder as it is usually due to stroke which is a highly prevalent condition. However, it does not appear that commonly in the exam.

Unless the other limb is being held in an abnormal position, if you are only asked to examine the upper or lower limbs you will only find a monoparesis (see below) and will be unaware of the presence of weakness in the ipsilateral limb not examined unless the examiner informs you.

Spastic monoparesis

If you are asked to examine only the upper or lower limb, remember that the finding of a monoparesis may be part of a hemiparesis (see above).

However, if it is a true monoparesis then it is likely to be due to either:

- a cerebral lesion affecting the contralateral motor cortex leg area (e.g. an anterior cerebral artery infarct), or
- an ipsilateral hemisection of the lower (thoracic/lumbar) spinal cord (Brown-Sequard syndrome), which may be accompanied by dissociated sensory loss: vibration and proprioception impairment ipsilateral to the monoparesis, and pain and temperature impairment contralaterally. Causes include trauma, tumours and demyelination.

Lower Motor Neurone Disorders

Summary of cases

- Anterior horn cell disorders — motor neurone disease and polio
- Radiculopathies and plexopathies
- Mononeuropathies — ulnar, median, radial, common peroneal and femoral nerves
- Mononeuritis multiplex
- Peripheral neuropathy
- Foot drop
- Absent ankle jerks and upgoing plantars

Anterior horn cell disorders

A unilateral or asymmetrical lower motor neurone syndrome without sensory features should raise the possibility of anterior horn cell disease.

If there are also upper motor neurone features (i.e. mixed UMN and LMN signs) then the diagnosis is likely to be motor neurone disease.

If there are no upper motor neurone features then the diagnosis is likely to be polio, the lower motor neurone only variant of MND (progressive muscular atrophy), or less commonly, a pure motor radiculopathy or multifocal motor neuropathy.

Old polio, however, should be relatively easily diagnosed as the patient needs to be of the correct age if born in the UK (i.e. born before widespread vaccination) or they need to be from an area in which polio remains (or has recently been) endemic. Furthermore, there may be substantial wasting in some cases and if acquired during childhood the limb may be shortened. In this case, it may be a 'spot diagnosis'.

Radiculopathies and plexopathies

These are relatively rare in the MRCP exam but should be thought of if the patient has unilateral or asymmetrical limb weakness with a lower motor neurone syndrome. Whilst syndromes may occasionally be pure motor, the presence of sensory signs in a dermatomal pattern may help in identifying that the disorder is at the level of the roots or plexus. Review Chapter 14 and also the dermatomal map in Chapter 1.

Mononeuropathies

These present with unilateral weakness and/or sensory disturbance in the distribution of the particular nerve.

Review Chapter 15 for the findings in the different common mononeuropathies — carpal tunnel syndrome (median nerve), ulnar nerve, radial nerve, common peroneal nerve and femoral nerve.

Mononeuritis multiplex

This presents with unilateral or asymmetrical weakness with a lower motor neurone syndrome. There are usually associated sensory features in the distribution of the particular nerves affected which help to localise the condition. The list of causes are given in Chapter 15 of Part 1.

Peripheral neuropathy

This is the most common of the lower motor neurone syndromes seen in the MRCP exam. The presence of distal symmetrical weakness with a lower motor syndrome indicates the presence of a motor neuropathy.

As discussed in Chapter 16 of Part 1, pure motor neuropathies have a small list of causes and therefore if you are allowed to carry on and perform a sensory examination, there is a large chance that there will also be a 'glove and stocking' sensory disturbance, i.e. a mixed sensorimotor neuropathy. The differential diagnosis of this is given in Chapter 16 of Part 1.

Clues to a particular diagnosis include the presence of pes cavus and clawed toes, which is likely to represent Charcot–Marie–Tooth disease. In this case, there may be severe distal wasting suggestive of long-standing disease. Be cautious about describing a patient with apparent high arches as having pes cavus as this is often overcalled by MRCP exam candidates. One way of testing for pes cavus is to put a flat object under the foot — daylight should not be visible under the arch normally.

Foot drop

This may be a case in the MRCP exam seen initially by watching the gait (which is high stepping on the side of the foot drop) or noticing a foot splint on inspection. The most common causes would be either a common peroneal nerve lesion or an L5 radiculopathy. Foot *inversion* is unaffected in common peroneal nerve lesions whilst it is weak in L5 root lesions (and *eversion* is weak in both). However, these two causes can be difficult to tell apart.

Also, there is a wider differential diagnosis which, thought of anatomically, may be in the upper motor neurone (which causes foot drop but is unlikely to be the only sign) or the lower motor neurone:

- *The anterior horn cell*, e.g. due to motor neurone disease
- *L5 nerve root*, e.g. due to a disc prolapse or space-occupying lesion
- *Lumbosacral plexopathy*
- *The sciatic/common peroneal/deep peroneal nerves*

Absent ankle jerks and upgoing plantars

This combination of signs is seen in motor neurone disease and this is the most likely diagnosis if there are widespread upper and lower motor neurone features.
Other causes of absent ankle jerks with upgoing plantars are:

- Vitamin B12 deficiency
- Friedreich's ataxia
- Syphilis
- Spinal cord lesions at the bottom of the cord, i.e. a lesion affecting the conus medullaris and surrounding roots

- Adrenomyeloneuropathy
- The presence of two separate disorders, e.g. spastic paraparesis and peripheral neuropathy

Neuromuscular Junction Disorders

Summary of cases

- Myasthenia gravis

Myasthenia gravis

This is rare in the limb examination in the MRCP exam as it is difficult to examine fatigability unless you are given the clue that there might be some. However, myasthenia gravis remains on the differential diagnosis of patients with symmetrical proximal weakness and particularly if there is accompanying bilateral ptosis and ophthalmoplegia.

Muscle Disorders

Summary of cases

- Proximal myopathy
- Myotonic dystrophy
- Muscular dystrophies

Proximal myopathy

This is relatively common in the MRCP exam with the inflammatory myopathies most commonly seen, i.e. polymyositis and dermatomyositis. The differential diagnosis of muscle disease is described in Chapter 18 of Part 1. If the patient has symmetrical proximal muscle weakness and/or wasting, look for other signs which may give the actual diagnosis, e.g. the presence of a heliotrope rash, photosensitive rash over sun-exposed areas and Gottron's papules suggest dermatomyositis. Features of endocrine disorders, e.g. acromegaly or hyperthyroidism (thyroid eye disease or tremor) may be present.

Myotonic dystrophy

This is a common 'spot diagnosis' in the MRCP exam. The features are described in detail in Chapter 18 of Part 1. Observation of the patient from the end of the bed will reveal myopathic facial features (bilateral ptosis, facial weakness and wasting) as well as frontal balding. On shaking the hand of the patient, they may have difficulty relaxing their grip. You may miss this as patients with myotonic dystrophy may not tightly grip your hand on shaking it, since they are aware of their own difficulties of relaxing the grip.

If you spot the diagnosis, go on to show the other features:

- Myotonia of grip — ask the patient to close their hands tightly into a fist and then release them as quickly as possible: there is delayed relaxation leading the patient to take a long time to open up their grip.
- Myotonia of eye opening — ask the patient to close their eyes tightly and then open them as quickly as possible: there is delayed opening of the eyes.
- Percussion myotonia of the thenar eminence — put your index finger over the thenar eminence and then hit it with your tendon hammer (one can also hit directly on to the thenar eminence): there is localised contraction (which may be seen as a dimple in the thenar eminence) which causes shortening of the muscle (in this case abductor pollicis brevis) and therefore movement at the joint (the thumb abducts).
- Cranial nerve territory examination may reveal facial weakness, ptosis, ophthalmoplegia and dysarthria.
- Unlike most other muscle diseases, in myotonic dystrophy weakness and wasting is distal in the upper limbs. Upper limb exam also reveals absent reflexes.

- Mention to the examiner the multisystem nature of the disorder (see the mnemonic ABCDE in Chapter 18 of Part 1) — you would want to examine the external genitalia in men to see if there is testicular atrophy, examine the eyes for cataracts, perform a cognitive examination, a cardiovascular examination (including seeing an ECG) looking for presence of a cardiomyopathy or a pacemaker (cardiac conduction defects), dipstick the urine for glucose (impaired glucose tolerance/diabetes) and perform a thyroid exam looking for a goitre.

Muscular dystrophies

These are relatively uncommon in the MRCP exam although they should be on the differential diagnosis of patients with proximal symmetrical weakness.

Patients may have wasting around the shoulder or limb girdle and the presence of pseudohypertrophy is suggestive of Becker or a limb girdle dystrophy (patients with Duchenne muscular dystrophy are usually in wheelchairs in their teens and therefore it would be unlikely that they would be seen in the MRCP exam).

Disorders that may be seen are:

- *Becker muscular dystrophy* — described in Chapter 18 of Part 1.
- *Limb girdle dystrophies* — these are a group of disorders connected by the clinical features of predominant shoulder and limb girdle weakness. They are either autosomal dominant or recessive inheritance and have multiple genetic causes. Pseudohypertrophy of the muscles is seen in some subtypes.
- *Facioscapulohumeral (FSH) dystrophy* — this is an autosomal dominant disorder with prominent facial weakness as well as bilateral winging of the scapulae (involvement of serratus anterior muscles) and difficulty with shoulder abduction. In the lower limbs, foot drop may be seen prior to involvement of the proximal muscles.
- *Oculopharyngeal muscular dystrophy (OPMD)* — this is an autosomal dominant disorder with ptosis, ophthalmoplegia,

dysphagia and weakness of the tongue. Proximal limb weakness may occur later in the illness.

Abnormal gait

There are a number of abnormal gaits which should be recognised, most of which have already been discussed. It should be noted that some patients do not have a 'classic' gait for many reasons (not the full signs seen in the condition, they are on treatment for it, etc.) and this makes identification of gait difficult in many patients. It is uncommon to be asked just to comment on the gait without any more of the exam except perhaps for a parkinsonian or ataxic gait.

- *Parkinsonian gait* — the festinant gait is seen in patients with parkinsonian syndromes. Patients have difficulty initiating gait and are stooped forward and have short, shuffling steps with decreased arm swing and difficulty turning. The rest tremor may become obvious in the hand whilst walking.
- *Ataxic gait* — patients with a cerebellar ataxia have a broad-based unsteady gait whilst patients with a sensory ataxia (due to proprioceptive sensory disturbance) have an unsteady gait that might be stamping in nature. Romberg's test distinguishes these — negative in cerebellar disease (patients almost equally unsteady with eyes open or closed) and positive in sensory ataxia (patients much more unsteady with the eyes closed).
- *Spastic gait* — this is seen in patients with spastic paraparesis or quadraparesis. The legs are stiff and are moved slowly. There may be scissoring, with the legs crossing each other.
- *Waddling gait* — patients with proximal symmetrical weakness, e.g. due to muscle disease, often have this kind of gait where the pelvis falls to the side of the leg being raised.
- *High-stepping gait* — this is seen in patients with foot drop (see above). The foot needs to be picked high up off the floor because of the weakness in dorsiflexion.
- *Hemiplegic gait* — this is seen in patients with a hemiparesis. The foot is swung around (circumducted) to stop it hitting the floor.

Part 3

Questions for Parts 1 and 2

Questions for Part 1

Question 1

A 68-year-old right-handed gentleman presents with a right parietal stroke. Which of the following cognitive symptoms is most likely?

A) Dyscalculia
B) Cortical blindness
C) Executive dysfunction
D) Visual neglect
E) Limb apraxia

Question 2

You are asked to see a 76-year-old woman on the ward who has become confused overnight. The nursing staff say she is fine in the day but is always confused at night. She often reaches out in front of her as if she is trying to touch something. The notes say her family have noticed some memory problems for the last year. She is difficult to examine but all her limbs seem stiff. What is the most likely diagnosis?

A) Alzheimer's disease
B) Frontotemporal dementia
C) Alcohol-induced dementia
D) Creutzfeldt–Jakob disease
E) Dementia with Lewy bodies

Question 3

A 25-year-old woman has just been diagnosed with generalised epilepsy. She is already on the combined oral contraceptive pill. Which of the following anti-epileptic drugs is an enzyme inducer and would cause her pill not to work?

A) Carbamazepine
B) Sodium valproate
C) Lorazepam
D) Gabapentin
E) Lamotrigine

Question 4

A 69-year-old man with known epilepsy presents to A+E feeling generally unwell. On measuring his urea and electrolytes, he was noted to have a sodium level of 120 mmol/l. Which anti-epileptic drug is most likely to have caused this?

A) Sodium valproate
B) Phenytoin
C) Carbamazepine
D) Lamotrigine
E) Gabapentin

Question 5

A 22-year-old woman presents with her first generalised tonic-clonic seizure. Her examination is normal. Routine blood tests, EEG and MRI brain scan are all normal. What is the most appropriate initial management?

A) Sodium valproate
B) Carbamazepine
C) No treatment
D) Lamotrigine
E) Levetiracetam

Question 6

Which of the following drugs are not commonly thought to be associated with idiopathic intracranial hypertension?

A) Tetracyclines
B) Isotretinoin
C) Nitrofurantoin
D) Oral contraceptive pill
E) Aminoglycosides

Question 7

A 79-year-old right-handed gentleman presents to A+E with an acute onset of speech production difficulties with drooping of the right side of his face and weakness of his right arm. Which arterial territory is likely to be affected?

A) Anterior cerebral artery
B) Middle cerebral artery
C) Posterior cerebral artery
D) Posterior inferior cerebellar artery
E) Basilar artery

Question 8

A 72-year-old right-handed gentleman presents to A+E with an acute onset of dizziness with sensory loss over the right side of his face and left arm and leg. On examination, his right pupil is smaller with a mild right ptosis. Which arterial territory is likely to be affected?

A) Left posterior inferior cerebellar artery
B) Left posterior cerebral artery
C) Right posterior cerebral artery
D) Right posterior inferior cerebellar artery
E) Right anterior cerebral artery

Question 9

A 62-year-old gentleman presents to A+E with a severe occipital headache for the last 16 hours. On examination, he has evidence of a stiff neck. His CT head is normal but a lumbar puncture reveals evidence of xanthochromia. Which of these medications would you start him on?

A) Propranolol
B) Ceftriaxone
C) Aciclovir
D) Nimodipine
E) Verapamil

Question 10

A 79-year-old right-handed gentleman presents to clinic with a six-month history of a stiff right arm which is interfering with his daily activities. His wife has noticed his voice has become quieter and his walking is slower than it was. Observing him, you notice his right hand is shaking at rest. Which drug would you start in this gentleman?

A) Levodopa
B) Propranolol
C) Selegiline
D) Entacapone
E) Lamotrigine

Question 11

A 55-year-old woman presents to clinic with a one-year history of shaking of both of her hands. This happens mostly when she is trying to carry something, e.g. a cup of tea, and is not there at rest. She thinks its because she has been more anxious since losing her job. She remembers her mother having similar problems. Apart from the tremor, the examination is normal. What medication would you start?

A) Levodopa
B) Ropinirole

C) Verapamil

D) Propranolol

E) Selegiline

Question 12

A 59-year-old man presents with a nine-month history of slower walking and dizziness on standing. On further questioning he has had erectile dysfunction for the last three years. On examination, he has a jerky postural tremor. What is the most likely diagnosis?

A) Progressive supranuclear palsy

B) Multiple system atrophy

C) Huntington's disease

D) Parkinson's disease

E) Wilson's disease

Question 13

A 33-year-old woman comes to the neurology outpatient clinic complaining of dizziness for the last few weeks and tingling on the left side of the body. She had had an episode a few years ago of blurred vision but was otherwise well. On examination, there is a relative afferent pupillary defect on the left as well as evidence of past-pointing and dysdiadochokinesia in her right arm. Which of the following two investigations will be most useful in coming to a diagnosis?

A) EMG

B) Serum CRP

C) Evoked potentials

D) MRI brain

E) Tensilon test

F) Nerve conduction studies

G) Serum autoantibodies

Question 14

A 73-year-old man is admitted after noticing that his walking was unsteady on getting out of bed in the morning. He has hypertension and type 2 diabetes mellitus and is on perindopril and metformin. On examination, there is jerky horizontal nystagmus. He also has some mild past-pointing in the left arm and difficulty in performing tandem walking. Where is the lesion most likely to be?

A) Foramen magnum
B) Right midbrain
C) Right cerebellum
D) Left internal capsule
E) Left cerebellum

Question 15

A 62-year-old man presents to A + E with acute onset visual disturbance. On examination, he has a left inferior homonymous quadrantanopia. Where is the lesion anatomically?

A) Left temporal lobe
B) Left parietal lobe
C) Optic chiasm
D) Right temporal lobe
E) Right parietal lobe

Question 16

A 58-year-old woman presents to outpatients as she has recently noticed her left pupil being smaller. On examination, she also has a mild left ptosis. Which of the following is unlikely to be a cause of her problem?

A) Apical lung tumour
B) Carotid dissection
C) Neck trauma
D) Lacunar stroke
E) Brainstem stroke

Question 17

A 64-year-old woman presents with an acutely painful left eye. On examination, the left pupil is dilated with no response to light, there is a ptosis and she has difficulty moving the eye apart from abduction and downgaze which remain intact. What is the most likely cause?

A) Diabetic cranial neuropathy
B) Posterior communicating artery aneurysm
C) Cavernous sinus thrombosis
D) Carotico-cavernous fistula
E) Superior orbital fissure syndrome

Question 18

A 55-year-old patient is brought to A+E after being found unconscious at home. You are asked to review the patient's neurological status three days following the admission. On examination, the patient has difficulty with upgaze and the pupils constrict with accommodation but do not react to light. Where is the lesion causing this clinical picture?

A) Bilateral watershed infarcts
B) Dorsal midbrain
C) Ventral pons
D) Lateral medulla
E) Cervico-medullary junction

Question 19

An 82-year-old woman presents with a slowly worsening history of intermittent sharp, shooting pains over the left side of her face for the last few months, made worse by eating. Examination of the cranial nerves is normal. What drug would you initially start this woman on?

A) Carbamazepine
B) Sodium valproate
C) Diazepam
D) Gabapentin
E) Lamotrigine

Question 20

A 33-year-old man presents with an acute onset of drooping of the left side of his face as well as vertigo and tinnitus. On examination, he has weakness of the whole left side of his face, affecting both upper and lower facial muscles. What is the most likely cause?

A) Bell's palsy
B) Brainstem stroke
C) Sarcoidosis
D) Multiple sclerosis
E) Ramsay Hunt syndrome

Question 21

A 41-year-old man presents with a three-day history of bilateral facial weakness. On examination, he has bilateral facial weakness worse on the left compared to the right, but an otherwise normal examination. He has recently returned from a trip to the East Coast of the US where he has been camping. Which test would be the most helpful in making the diagnosis?

A) Anti-GQ1b antibody
B) Nerve conduction studies
C) ACE
D) Borrelia serology
E) Parotid ultrasound

Question 22

A 46-year-old woman presents with an acute history of double vision. On examination, there is evidence of a complete ophthalmo-plegia. The limb examination is normal apart from an inability to elicit any reflexes. She is also unsteady walking. Which antibody is likely to be positive?

A) Anti-GM1
B) Anti-voltage gated potassium channel
C) Anti-ACh receptor
D) Anti-GQ1b
E) Anti-voltage gated calcium channel

Question 23

A 45-year-old woman with known hypothyroidism presents with a few months' history of difficulty walking. She has been well, apart from some recent fatigue. On examination, she has increased tone in the legs bilaterally with weakness of the flexor muscles and pathologically brisk reflexes. Sensory exam reveals abnormal proprioception and vibration to the hip but normal pinprick. Which test is most likely to be abnormal?

A) CRP
B) Blood film
C) ANA
D) VDRL
E) HTLV-1

Question 24

A 50-year-old woman with a known quadraparesis following a teenage horseriding accident became worse on her legs over a three-month period. Examination reveals a spastic quadraparesis, but with greater weakness than when last examined as well as sensory loss to pinprick over the shoulders and lateral aspects of both arms. What is the most likely cause?

A) Spinal abscess
B) Spinal haematoma
C) Cervical spondylosis
D) Syringomyelia
E) Anterior spinal artery infarction

Question 25

A 66-year-old man presents with a two-month history of weakness of his right leg and a one-month history of left wrist drop. On examination, he has wasting and fasciculations in the right leg and left forearm with weakness of hip flexion bilaterally, brisk reflexes thoughout and upgoing plantars. The rest of the neurological examination is normal. What is the most likely diagnosis?

A) Vitamin B12 deficiency
B) Motor neurone disease
C) Multifocal motor neuropathy
D) Multiple sclerosis
E) Friedreich's ataxia

Question 26

A 42-year-old man complains of a two-week history of leg weakness and sensory disturbance. He also reports having had an episode of visual blurring in the left eye, five years ago, lasting a few days. Examination of the cranial nerve territory and upper limb is normal. In the legs, tone is normal but there is weakness in hip and knee flexion on the left. Vibration sense is absent at the metatarsophalangeal joint on the left with a couple of errors on joint position testing distally also on the left. In the right leg there is no weakness but pin prick sensation is not as sharp as in the left leg. The reflexes are brisk in the left leg but normal elsewhere. Where is the lesion?

A) Cauda equina
B) Right cervical cord
C) Conus medullaris
D) Left thoracic cord
E) Left midbrain

Question 27

A 19-year-old man presents with a twelve-month history of difficulty walking and a four-month history of abdominal pain and fatigue. On examination, he has increased tone in both legs with weakness of the flexors bilaterally and pathologically brisk reflexes at the knees but absent reflexes at the ankles and upgoing plantars.

Blood tests show a sodium level of 120 mmol/l and a potassium level of 5.9 mmol/l. What is the most likely diagnosis?

A) Vitamin B12 deficiency
B) Motor neurone disease
C) Adrenoleukodystrophy
D) Multiple sclerosis
E) Friedreich's ataxia

Question 28

A 59-year-old man presents with a three-month history of back pain and a feeling of weakness in the left leg. On examination, he has normal tone, weakness of knee extension and ankle dorsiflexion, a reduced left knee jerk but preserved right knee jerk and both ankle jerks. There is a patch of sensory loss over the medial part of his left shin. Which nerve root is affected?

A) L1
B) L2
C) L3
D) L4
E) L5

Question 29

A 29-year-old woman presents with a three-month history of progressive weakness in the legs with numbness over her legs and trunk. On examination, she has increased tone in the legs, weakness particularly of the flexors as well as brisk knee and ankle reflexes. Sensory disturbance is in both legs and the trunk with a level at the nipples. At what level in the spinal cord is the lesion likely to be?

A) C4
B) C8
C) T4
D) T8
E) T10

Question 30

A 35-year-old gentleman presents to A+E after a motorcycle accident. His right arm is weak with difficulty in shoulder abduction, elbow extension and wrist extension. He also has sensory loss over two areas, one over the outer aspect of the upper arm and one in a small patch over the dorsal aspect of his hand above the thumb. Where in the brachial plexus is the lesion likely to be?

A) Lateral cord
B) Upper trunk
C) Lower trunk
D) Posterior cord
E) Medial cord

Question 31

A 76-year-old man complains of weakness in his right hand. He has weakness of finger abduction, finger adduction and thumb abduction. There were no other positive findings on examination. Where is the lesion?

A) Median nerve
B) C8 root
C) T1 root
D) Upper brachial plexus
E) Ulnar nerve

Question 32

You are asked to see a 63-year-old gentleman on the cardiology ward who presents with difficulty mobilising due to right leg weakness. He underwent a primary angioplasty after an anterior myocardial infarction three days previously. On examination, he has weakness of knee extension on the right. His knee reflex was present only with reinforcement on the right but the other reflexes were normal. Sensation to pinprick over the anterior thigh on the right was subjectively impaired. What is the most likely cause for his weakness?

A) Left anterior cerebral artery infarct
B) Anterior spinal artery occlusion
C) Right L2 lesion
D) Femoral neuropathy
E) Cauda equina syndrome

Question 33

A 36-year-old gentleman has been complaining of hand weakness after fracturing his elbow a few weeks earlier. Weakness in which of the following muscles would suggest this is not purely an ulnar neuropathy?

A) Abductor digiti minimi
B) 1st dorsal interosseous
C) Adductor pollicis
D) 3rd lumbrical
E) Flexor pollicis brevis

Question 34

Which of the following disorders is caused by excess phytanic acid?

A) Tangier disease
B) Refsum's disease
C) Maple syrup urine disease
D) Laurence–Moon–Bardet–Biedl syndrome
E) Kearns–Sayre syndrome

Question 35

A 48-year-old man presents with a feeling of generalised weakness shortly after discharge from hospital for treatment of an infection. On examination, he has a fatigable weakness of shoulder abduction. Which drug might he have been given during his stay in hospital?

A) Imipenem
B) Ceftriaxone
C) Amoxicillin
D) Trimethoprim
E) Ciprofloxacin

Question 36

A 59-year-old man presents with a six-month history of difficulty opening jars and walking up stairs. On examination he has weakness in the finger extensors in the upper limb and in the quadriceps in the lower limb. What is the most likely diagnosis?

A) Myotonic dystrophy
B) Steroid-induced myopathy
C) Alcohol-induced myopathy
D) Inclusion body myositis
E) Polymyositis

Question 37

Which of the following disorders is a trinucleotide repeat disorder?

A) Multiple system atrophy
B) Spinobulbar muscular atrophy
C) Duchenne muscular dystrophy
D) Primary lateral sclerosis
E) Limb girdle muscular dystrophy

Question 38

Which of the following is an X-linked disorder?

A) Huntington's disease
B) Duchenne muscular dystrophy
C) DRPLA

D) Familial Alzheimer's disease
E) MELAS

Question 39

Which of the following is not a feature of type 1 neurofibromatosis?

A) Café au lait spots
B) Axillary freckles
C) Lisch nodules
D) Periungual fibromas
E) Optic nerve gliomas

Question 40

A 43-year-old man presents with sudden onset right hemiparesis and speech production impairment. On examination, he has weakness of the right side of the face, arm and leg with brisk reflexes on the right. Whilst examining him, you note some small, dark papular skin lesions over the lower trunk and tops of the legs. Which enzyme deficiency is this man likely to have?

A) Alpha-galactosidase
B) Glucocerebrosidase
C) Arylsulfatase A
D) Sphingomyelinase
E) Alpha-L-iduronidase

Questions for Part 2

Question 1

A 67-year-old woman presents with a two-month history of rapidly progressive cognitive decline and jerking movements in the limbs. Which of the following tests is most likely to be helpful in the diagnosis?

A) Genetic testing
B) CSF 14-3-3
C) Neuropsychology testing
D) CSF oligoclonal bands
E) CT brain scan

Question 2

A 37-year-old woman is seen in clinic. She has been accused of unprofessional behaviour at work and was referred to a psychiatrist by her GP who treated her for depression with citalopram. There is no previous medical history of note, although she admits to occasional use of cocaine and ecstasy and smokes ten cigarettes daily. Her only medication is the oral contraceptive pill. Her mother is well, although she has had no contact with her father for many years as their relationship broke down when she became pregnant. She remembers he had been suffering from depression as his father had recently died with dementia. On examination, she has irregular fidgety movements of the face and hands but the rest of the examination is normal. What is the most likely diagnosis?

A) Recreational drug use
B) Huntington's disease
C) Depression
D) Oral contraceptive pill use
E) Creutzfeldt–Jakob disease

Question 3

A 54-year-old man is brought to A+E after being found with a reduced level of consciousness. His GCS is 8 (M4, V2, E2). On arrival, he appears dehydrated and his blood glucose is 2.3. He is given oxygen, intravenous fluids and 50 ml of 50% dextrose. His GCS quickly improves to 14 (M6, V5, E3). He is admitted and treated for pneumonia. The following morning he is noted to be confused and falls on trying to get out of bed. Examination is difficult because of his confusion but there is restriction of abduction in both eyes with nystagmus on bilateral gaze although the rest of the neurological examination is normal. What is the most likely cause of his deterioration?

A) Acute confusional state secondary to his pneumonia
B) Subdural haematoma with raised intracranial pressure
C) Hypoxic-ischaemic encephalopathy
D) Wernicke's encephalopathy
E) Brainstem stroke

Question 4

A 37-year-old Bolivian cleaner has been referred to the Neurology outpatient clinic after collapsing at work. He reports three previous episodes of collapse at work in the last year. During the most recent episode he awoke on the floor with no clear recollection of why he lost consciousness. He had been incontinent of urine and on one previous occasion had had a painful tongue. His MRI scan is abnormal with multiple white matter lesions. What is the most likely cause of this gentleman's seizures?

A) Hippocampal sclerosis
B) Toxoplasmosis
C) Venous sinus thrombosis
D) Glioblastoma multiforme
E) Cysticercosis

Question 5

A 36-year-old lady has a diagnosis of temporal lobe seizures with secondary generalisation, made five years ago. She has tried many anti-epileptic drugs, none of which have made any difference to her seizure frequency. You suspect she may be suffering from a non-epileptic attack disorder. Which of the following features would not be in keeping with such a diagnosis?

A) Rapid post-ictal orientation
B) Eyes firmly shut during attack
C) Lateral tongue biting
D) Absence of cyanosis
E) Seizures commonly lasting 30 minutes

Question 6

A 60-year-old gentleman presents to the A+E department with a left-sided headache which came on fairly rapidly earlier in the afternoon. The headache is retro-orbital and also affects the left side of the neck. On examination, he has a left-sided partial ptosis and the left pupil appears slightly smaller than the right but is reactive to light and accommodates. The rest of the examination is normal. What is the most likely diagnosis?

A) Left carotid dissection
B) Left anterior cerebral artery infarct
C) Venous sinus thrombosis
D) Left frontal haemorrhage
E) Senile miosis and cervical spondylosis

Question 7

A 76-year-old gentleman presents with sudden onset word-finding difficulty. His spontaneous speech is full of neologisms (made-up words) and does not make sense. What is the most likely diagnosis?

A) Right middle cerebral artery infarct
B) Left posterior cerebral artery infarct
C) Left middle cerebral artery infarct
D) Left anterior cerebral artery infarct
E) Right anterior cerebral artery infarct

Question 8

A 38-year-old woman had recently been diagnosed with migraine by her GP. Over the last week her headache has become gradually more severe and persistent, requiring daily analgesia. She is brought to A+E by concerned colleagues. Whilst in A+E she has a generalised tonic-clonic seizure. She is apyrexial but is drowsy and confused with marked papilloedema. Neurological examination is otherwise normal. A CT scan is normal and a CSF examination is performed. Her opening pressure is 31 cm H_2O. CSF cell count, glucose and protein are normal. What is the most appropriate treatment?

A) Aspirin
B) Low molecular weight heparin
C) Ceftriaxone
D) Aciclovir
E) Sumatriptan

Question 9

A 28-year-old lady presents with a history of episodic retro-orbital left-sided severe headaches associated with nausea and phonophobia. Over the last six months these headaches have been largely replaced by a more generalised headache present on three to four days every week. These improve a little with analgesia, only to deteriorate before the next analgesic dose is required. She is using 30 mg of codeine three times a day when she has the headache. What is the likely diagnosis of her new headache?

A) Medication overuse headache
B) Cluster headache
C) Tension headache
D) Idiopathic intracranial hypertension
E) Paroxysmal hemicrania

Question 10

A 34-year-old man presents with a headache after clearing his garden a week ago. His headache is worse towards the end of the day after standing up for a long period, and is better on lying down. There is some improvement in the headache with caffeine. He has no history of headaches. His neurological examination is normal. What is the likely cause of his headache?

A) Glioblastoma multiforme
B) Low pressure headache
C) Migraine
D) Cluster headache
E) Idiopathic intracranial hypertension

Question 11

A 37-year-old gentleman presents to A+E having developed severe right periorbital headaches over the last ten days. The pain lasts for an hour during which time he walks around, at times hitting his head on the wall to seek relief from the pain. The right eye becomes red during these episodes and this is accompanied by a mild ptosis. What would be the best acute treatment for the headaches?

A) Verapamil
B) Aspirin
C) Topiramate
D) Oxygen
E) Heparin

Question 12

A 36-year-old right-handed gentleman with known HIV presents to A+E with a one-month history of headache and feeling generally unwell. A lumbar puncture reveals the following: white cells 50 (90% lymphocytes), red cells 2, glucose 2.5 mmol/l (serum 6.9 mmol/l), protein 2.2 g/dl. Which two further tests would be most useful in helping to get to a diagnosis?

A) Nerve conduction studies
B) CSF oligoclonal bands
C) CSF Ziehl–Neelsen stain
D) EEG
E) CSF xanthochromia
F) Visual evoked potentials
G) CSF India ink stain

Question 13

A patient recently underwent neurosurgery for cervical cord compression but is readmitted after becoming unwell with headache and confusion. A CT scan of the brain is normal. CSF examination reveals the following: white cells 35 (90% neutrophils), red cells 7, glucose 2.2 mmol/l (serum 6 mmol/l), protein 0.92 g/dl. Which of the following is the most likely cause for this presentation?

A) Lymphomatous infiltration of the meninges
B) HSV encephalitis
C) TB meningitis
D) Bacterial meningitis
E) Viral meningitis

Question 14

A 65-year-old man presents with a one-year history of behavioural change consisting of increasing disinhibition. He has started to fall backwards regularly. On examination, he has axial rigidity and slowed downward saccadic eye movements. The rest of the neuro-logical examination was normal. What is the most likely diagnosis?

A) Huntington's disease
B) Spinocerebellar ataxia
C) Progressive supranuclear palsy
D) Multiple system atrophy
E) Dentatorubropallidoluysian atrophy

Question 15

A 27-year-old woman is readmitted 12 hours after being discharged by the Gynaecology team. She is 12 weeks pregnant and was an inpatient for three days being treated for hyperemesis gravidarum. She presents with trismus, preventing her from speaking, retrocollis and upwards deviation of the eyes. Which of the following is the first-line treatment for her condition?

A) IM Risperidone
B) IV Procyclidine
C) PO Diazepam
D) PO Sinemet
E) IV Phenytoin

Question 16

A 39-year-old man is brought in to A+E. He is confused but is known to have schizophrenia for which he is on fluphenazine. He was pyrexial at 38 degrees Celsius as well as being hypotensive and tachycardic with a respiratory rate of 25 breaths per minute and sat-urations of 97%. On examination, he was mildly confused and sweating profusely. He had marked stiffness of all four limbs but the rest of the examination is normal. Which two drugs would you use to treat this problem?

A) Prednisolone
B) Bromocriptine
C) Ceftriaxone

D) Sodium valproate
E) Clarithromycin
F) Aciclovir
G) Dantrolene
H) Topiramate

Question 17

A 17-year-old boy presents with progressive difficulty in walking. His legs feel stiff and he is no longer able to play football as he is repeatedly tripping. His aunt had similar symptoms, occurring in her early twenties. His paternal grandfather, an only child, also had life-long difficulties walking and died of a myocardial infarction aged 59. On examination, he is mildly dysarthric. There is pes cavus bilaterally and tone is increased in both legs. Power is decreased in the lower limbs with absent knee and ankle jerks but extensor plantars. Pinprick sensation is intact but there is a loss of vibration and joint position sense distally. He is unsteady on tandem walking. What is the most likely diagnosis?

A) Charcot–Marie–Tooth disease type 1
B) Hereditary spastic paraparesis
C) Multiple sclerosis
D) Friedreich's ataxia
E) Abetalipoproteinaemia

Question 18

A 56-year-old gentleman presents to the emergency clinic with a painless loss of vision affecting the left eye, occurring over the last 24 hours. On examination, visual acuity is 6/6 on the right but 6/60 on the left, which does not correct with a pin hole. His peripheral visual fields are intact to confrontation. His pupils are equal but on the swinging flashlight test the left eye dilates on shining a light in that eye. Fundoscopy reveals no abnormalities on the right but the left disc appears swollen. His CRP is 13 and ESR 21. What is the most likely cause of this man's visual loss?

A) Giant cell arteritis
B) Optic neuritis
C) Ischaemic optic neuropathy
D) Optic nerve compression
E) Retinal detachment

Question 19

A 22-year-old woman presents after her new partner has noticed that her left pupil is larger than the right. She is otherwise well with no visual symptoms. Examination reveals the left pupil to react sluggishly to light. The pupil does constrict when accommodating but this response is slow and persists after refocusing on a distant object. Her limb examination is normal except for the reflexes which appear symmetrically diminished. What is the diagnosis?

A) Argyll Robertson pupil
B) Partial 3rd nerve palsy
C) Right sided Horner's syndrome
D) Idiopathic anisocoria
E) Holmes–Adie syndrome

Question 20

A 33-year-old woman presents two months after an episode of diplopia which has now resolved. Her symptoms developed over 48 hours and she noted mild diplopia when looking to the right. Her symptoms occasionally return for a very short period of time after a hot bath. She is otherwise well. Examination reveals normal pupillary reactions and size. There is a full range of motion on testing eye movements but the left eye appears to adduct more slowly on asking the patient to quickly look to the right. This is associated with some subtle nystagmus in the abducted right eye at the same time. What is the diagnosis?

A) Parinaud's syndrome
B) Partial left 3rd nerve palsy
C) Supranuclear gaze palsy

D) Internuclear ophthalmoplegia
E) 6th nerve palsy

Question 21

A 48-year-old woman presents with diplopia. She reports that three weeks ago she developed a 'whooshing' in her right ear which has persisted. Since then, she feels her eye is swollen and over the last week she reports diplopia which is worse when looking to the left hand side. She has no relevant past medical history but her mother developed glaucoma in her 50s. On examination, there is proptosis and conjunctival injection affecting the right eye which is deviated to the right. Visual acuity is normal. The pupils are both reactive to light but there is an anisocoria with the right measuring 7 mm compared to 5 mm on the left. There is diplopia in the primary position which is worst when looking to the left-hand side. On looking left the right eye adducts poorly. There is also some impairment of upgaze and downgaze in the right eye. There are no other abnormalities on the rest of the cranial nerve territory or limb examination. The auditory canals and tympanic membranes appear normal. What is the most likely cause for this lady's presentation?

A) Pituitary apoplexy
B) Carotico-cavernous fistula
C) Cavernous sinus thrombosis
D) Right midbrain haemorrhage
E) Orbital cellulitis

Question 22

A 29-year-old lady presents with diplopia in all directions of gaze. This has developed gradually over the last six weeks. She is otherwise well, although she has not had a period for the last four months. On examination, there is a partial ptosis of the right eye and a mild anisocoria with the right pupil slightly larger than the left. Visual acuity is decreased in the right eye. There is restriction of all movements in the right eye maximal for abduction. What is the likely diagnosis?

A) Idiopathic intracranial hypertension
B) Thyroid eye disease
C) Myasthenia gravis
D) Sphenoid wing meningioma
E) Multiple sclerosis

Question 23

A 67-year-old man presents complaining of tinnitus in the right ear which has gradually progressed over three months. His hearing has become slightly impaired over a number of years which he has always attributed to normal aging. On examination, he has a diminished corneal reflex on the right-hand side but otherwise trigeminal function is normal. Weber's test lateralises to the left-hand side. The rest of the examination is normal. What is the most likely cause for this gentleman's findings?

A) Vestibular schwannoma
B) Trigeminal neurofibroma
C) Pontine glioma
D) Meniere's disease
E) Middle ear infection

Question 24

You are asked to review an 83-year-old lady who was admitted to the general medical ward. She fell over three days ago and hit her head. She does not remember the episode very well but since then has had multiple episodes of dizziness, particularly on turning her head to the left, and is now confined to bed where her symptoms are tolerable. She is hypertensive and hypercholesterolaemic but has had no previous strokes. Routine neurological examination reveals no abnormalities but her dizziness is recreated by lying her down flat and turning her head to the left. What is the most likely diagnosis?

A) Viral labyrinthitis
B) Meniere's disease
C) Brainstem infarct

D) Vestibular schwannoma
E) Benign paroxysmal positional vertigo

Question 25

A 71-year-old man presents to the clinic with dysarthria. Which of the following features would be in keeping with a bulbar palsy rather than a pseudobulbar palsy?

A) Nasal speech
B) Brisk jaw jerk
C) Emotional incontinence
D) Brisk gag reflex
E) Slow tongue movements

Question 26

A 56-year-old woman presents with a one-year history of hearing impairment in the left ear associated with the feeling that she could hear her heart beating in her ear. Over the last nine months she had also developed dysphagia, particularly for liquids. On examination, she had a hoarse voice, wasting of the sternocleidomastoid and trapezius on the left and a decreased gag reflex. Rinne's test showed air conduction was better than bone conduction on the right whilst bone conduction was better than air conduction on the left and Weber's test lateralised to the left ear. What is the most likely diagnosis?

A) Syringobulbia
B) Myasthenia gravis
C) Vestibular schwannoma
D) Motor neurone disease
E) Glomus jugulare tumour

Question 27

A 45-year-old man presents with a three-year history of progressive difficulty walking. He has been living in the UK for three years but is originally from Jamaica. His legs are stiff and he has had several falls. He has urinary urgency associated with hesitancy and a sense of incomplete voiding. He complains of a diffuse burning pain in the legs. He is systemically well. What is the most likely diagnosis?

A) Parasagittal meningioma
B) Metastatic prostate cancer
C) Adrenoleukodystrophy
D) Transverse myelitis
E) HTLV-1 infection

Question 28

A 19-year-old man presents with a one-year history of bilateral foot drop. On examination, he has distal symmetrical weakness as well as some wasting of the distal muscles and clawing of the toes. All of the reflexes were depressed throughout and both coordination and sensory examinations were normal. What is the most likely diagnosis?

A) Syringomyelia
B) Charcot–Marie–Tooth disease
C) Motor neurone disease
D) Cervical spondylosis
E) Polymyositis

Question 29

A 56-year-old man presents to the Endocrinology outpatients where he is given a diagnosis of type 2 diabetes. He has been living in the UK for the last five years having been born in Bangladesh. He has had difficulty walking since early childhood. On examination, he is noted to have a small wasted right leg with globally reduced power and absent reflexes in the affected leg. The sensory examination is normal. What is the most likely diagnosis?

A) Diabetic amyotrophy
B) Diabetic polyneuropathy
C) Cerebral palsy

D) Poliomyelitis
E) Spinal muscular atrophy

Question 30

A 37-year-old factory worker presents to you with a one-week history of severe right shoulder and neck pain. He is taking maximal doses of paracetamol and ibuprofen with little benefit. You prescribe opioid-based analgesics. He returns four weeks later with little pain but he complains of shoulder weakness affecting abduction. On examination, you note mild winging of the scapula. What is the most likely diagnosis?

A) C4 radiculopathy
B) C5 radiculopathy
C) Brachial neuritis
D) Cervical rib
E) Neoplastic infiltration of brachial plexus

Question 31

A 27-year-old woman presents with a ten-day history of lower back and buttock pain. In the last five days she has developed a diminished desire to micturate and defecate and when she does she feels the need to strain. She also complains that toilet paper feels strange over the vulval and perianal area. On examination, she has slight difficulty with standing on her tiptoes but power on the bed is full throughout. Tone is normal. Reflexes are present but the right ankle jerk requires reinforcement. Plantars are flexor. An urgent MRI scan of the spine is requested and reveals the cause of her symptoms. Which of the following is most likely?

A) Demyelination of the cervical cord
B) Central disc prolapse at S1
C) Infiltrative mass from the cervix
D) Conus medullaris lesion
E) Thoracic syrinx

Question 32

A 36-year-old lady presents complaining of nocturnal hand pain. Which of the following conditions are not associated with carpal tunnel syndrome?

A) Acromegaly
B) Hypothyroidism
C) Pregnancy
D) Rheumatoid arthritis
E) Addison's disease

Question 33

A 43-year-old man presents with wasting of the left hand and a burning pain in the right hand. He was diagnosed with asthma five years ago and uses salmeterol and fluticasone inhalers twice a day. He was admitted for an acute asthma attack earlier in the year requiring nebulisers and oral steroids. On examination, he has mild expiratory wheeze. There is wasting of the first dorsal interosseous in the left hand with weakness of finger abduction whilst in the right hand there is mild weakness of the abductor pollicis brevis and decreased sensation in the thumb and index finger. Routine blood tests reveal a moderate eosinophilia, an ESR of 47 and a positive ANCA. What is the most likely diagnosis?

A) Sarcoidosis
B) Polyarteritis nodosa
C) Churg-Strauss vasculitis
D) Diabetes
E) HIV

Question 34

A 27-year-old man is admitted to hospital with a one-week history of difficulty climbing stairs at work. He was treated by his GP with antibiotics for a fever and cough two weeks ago which resolved with treatment. On examination, he has bilateral foot drop but also more proximal weakness in the legs. He is areflexic but there is no sensory loss. His upper limb and cranial nerve territory examinations are normal. What is the most likely diagnosis?

A) Botulism
B) Guillain–Barré syndrome
C) Porphyria
D) Myasthenia gravis
E) Polymyositis

Question 35

A 23-year-old woman developed an acute onset of weakness in her legs shortly after returning from a holiday in Spain. Over the next few days she developed worsening weakness in the legs and also weakness in both arms. She attends A+E. What is the most important initial investigation?

A) FBC
B) Peak flow
C) Vital capacity
D) Serum potassium
E) ABG

Question 36

A 32-year-old man presents with an acute onset of weakness in the legs. His partner has also noted him to be confused and agitated today. He has been diagnosed with irritable bowel syndrome after several episodes of unexplained abdominal pain, one of which required hospital admission. Examination reveals distal limb weakness with areflexia. The sensory examination is difficult to interpret given his confusion but appears grossly intact. What is the likely diagnosis?

A) Guillain–Barré syndrome
B) Lead poisoning
C) Botulism

D) Porphyria

E) Multifocal motor neuropathy

Question 37

A 55-year-old woman has been complaining of weakness in her hands and feet with some loss of sensation distally. Nerve conduction studies showed reduced conduction velocity but normal amplitude. Which disorder is the most likely cause?

A) Diabetic neuropathy

B) Paraproteinaemic neuropathy

C) Vasculitic neuropathy

D) Paraneoplastic neuropathy

E) Drug-induced neuropathy

Question 38

A 66-year-old man presents with a two-month history of feeling weak and tired with difficulty getting out of his chair. He had been constipated for the last month and in the week before seeing you he had had difficulty swallowing. He used to smoke 40 cigarettes per day for many years and drank around 30 units of alcohol per week. Limb examination revealed mild proximal weakness in all four limbs as well as decreased reflexes throughout. However, the reflexes returned to normal after exercising that muscle group. What test would confirm the diagnosis?

A) Acetlycholine receptor antibodies

B) Nerve conduction studies

C) CK

D) Nerve biopsy

E) MRI spine

Question 39

A 41-year-old man presents with progressive difficulty in climbing stairs as well as difficulty at work as a carpenter with manipulation of tools. He reports no other neurological symptoms but that his work colleagues refer to him as 'sleepy' on account of his facial appearance. He is married but has no children as he and his wife have not been able to conceive. His immediate family are well but a paternal uncle and his grandfather were both said to have had a 'nerve disorder'. On examination, he has bilateral ptosis, weakness in the hands and feet but the rest of the examination is normal. What is the most likely diagnosis?

A) Graves' disease
B) Myasthenia gravis
C) Leber's optic atrophy
D) Myotonic dystrophy
E) Freidreich's ataxia

Question 40

A 22-year-old man presents to A+E with rapidly progressive weakness, developing over two hours following a large family meal to celebrate the Chinese New Year. He is globally weak, unable to move at all with just a flicker of power in the limbs, with absent reflexes, but speaking and swallowing are normal as is sensation. Cranial nerves are normal. By the next morning he is completely better. What is the diagnosis?

A) Porphyria
B) Hypokalaemic periodic paralysis
C) Psychogenic weakness
D) Guillain–Barré syndrome
E) Myasthenia gravis

Answers to Questions

All questions are based on disorders discussed in the main text. Refer to the particular section to learn more about the condition.

Part 1

1. D
2. E
3. A
4. C
5. C
6. E
7. B
8. D
9. D
10. A
11. D
12. B
13. C and D
14. E
15. E
16. D
17. B
18. B
19. A
20. E
21. D
22. D

23. B
24. D
25. B
26. D
27. C
28. D
29. C
30. D
31. C
32. D
33. E
34. B
35. E
36. D
37. B
38. B
39. D
40. A

Part 2

1. B
2. B
3. D
4. E
5. C
6. A
7. C
8. B
9. A
10. B
11. D
12. C and G
13. D
14. C
15. B

16. B and G
17. D
18. C
19. E
20. D
21. B
22. D
23. A
24. E
25. A
26. E
27. E
28. B
29. D
30. C
31. B
32. E
33. C
34. B
35. C
36. D
37. B
38. B
39. D
40. B

Index

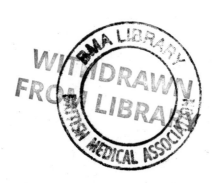